The Healthy Dude Book

Trisha Stewart

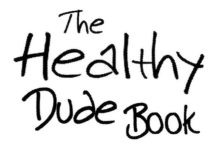

The Essential Guide for Men of All Ages who want to Eat Right, Get in Shape and Stay Healthy! Including the famous 30 day detox plan and full flexible workout regime.

By Trisha Stewart

Visit us on the web at:
www.HealthyDudeBook.com
www.TrishaStewart.com
www.ChristinMcdowell.com

ISBN 978-0-9816846-1-1

Other books by Trisha Stewart include:
    Healthy Tart
    Healthy Idol
    Healthy Bunch Cookbook

Books by Christin McDowell
    Healthy Fitness Central

Dedications

To my late Father, whose drive and ambition inspired and encouraged me to become an authority in the field of nutrition and wellness.

Acknowledgements

Thanks to my teams of healthy lifestyles devotees in the preparation of this book. The team includes Chris, Mavis, Jo, Mike, Mary, Christin and Phil.

Maude Lebowski:	*What do you do for recreation?*
The Dude:	*Oh, the usual. I bowl. Drive around.*
	The occasional acid flashback.

The Big Lebowski

Contents

The Healthy Dude Book

Introduction

This book is written for men of all ages who want to know how to take real care of themselves; who want to look great till late and be fit and healthy enough to enjoy life to the utmost!

We are going to discover how to get fit, yes really fit! Whether in the gym, on the track or just running around the block with some other work thrown in; we will make it as simple as you like or as much of a challenge - whatever you're up for.

Worried about belly fat? We'll show you the best way to combat this ugly problem and how to improve your upper body physique.

Ensure your leg muscles are strong and up to the work of carrying you around without pressure on the joints.

The focus will be on eating foods that will give your body everything it needs to stay at the correct weight, maintain lean muscle tissue, re-build and repair the body cells, take care of the hormones, the immune system and more.

We've included the ultimate 30 day detox and revitalize plan. This will take you through all the steps you need to kick start your journey to a complete healthy lifestyle. Included are recipes, planned menus, shopping lists and other information –

also supported by the 24/7 www.trishastewart.com full resource centre.

Find out how those all important hormones, (other than Testosterone!), are affected by what you do, what you eat and how you operate in your daily life. Infertility, impotence, motility, lack of libido or sex drive; and those issues that affect far more of you men than you imagine.

Stress: that ubiquitous but never easy to resolve issue. What can you do about it? How are you sleeping? Are you waking un-refreshed? Falling asleep on the couch after work? Sleeping in at weekends instead of being out with the family or friends? I will show you how to get the best out of life and get on top of the stress!

What about outwardly ageing? Don't tell me there's a man out there who doesn't truly care about that! Well, I know that's not you because you're reading this book!! Yes, of course men care! Why are there so many skin products and beauty salons especially for men? But I think that's great!!! I am one of many women really delighted that men are encouraged to make the very best of their appearance. They say beauty is only skin deep but I know the skin will show all; so if it's not looking good it will tell a lot about the deeper man.

Disease and ill health – What parts of your body do you need to check out? Where and when should you get tested?

Learn about prostate problems, depression, heart disease, high cholesterol, high blood pressure, diabetes, skin problems, bowel diseases and more. How to prevent and even cure certain diseases! I'll show you how to overcome a multitude of health challenges by using natural remedies: instead of drugs.

Digestive health: Too many people don't understand the workings (or importance) of this crucial system!!! IBS, constipation, indigestion, colitis, diverticulitis, ulcers, bowel cancer and more! Yes, these do affect you men, although you may think you are unique! We ALL have the same basic functions! I am going to show you how to prevent these health challenges - or if you already have them, how to get rid of them.

Goal setting and rewards for attaining those goals. Let's set some simple goals to get you motivated, and then work out some exciting rewards for when you reach your ultimate goal.

This book together with Healthy Fitness Central, Healthy Bunch Cookbook and the trishastewart.com website will be all you need to attain the healthy lifestyle you have always wanted.

Healthy Dude - Chapter 1

Adam was a Dude...Dudes live in Eden

Okay, I know you're probably thinking, "Trisha – what are you talking about? Adam...Eden...I just want to lose a few pounds, maybe lower my blood pressure. What's all this?" Well, let me explain. I introduced the concept of living in "Eden" in my first book, **Healthy Tart**. And, if living in Eden is good for the Eves out there, it's good for all you Adams as well. Now, before you get too concerned...I am NOT talking about religion or a faith-based type of Eden. I'm simply referring to a place to live that's more ideal...better suited to being and staying healthy. I think you'd agree with me that our world is far from the clean, pure, pollution free place it once was. In fact, the world isn't even as clean as it was when you were a kid. And, it seems to be getting a bit worse every day. Something's got to change...even if it's just you!!

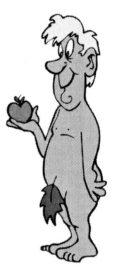

"We can't solve problems by using the same kind of thinking we used when we created them." - **Albert Einstein**

Einstein was really onto something here...and you've probably heard a variation of this thought in different forms. But, the bottom line is if you aren't where you'd like to be (and for purposes of this book I'm focusing on your health) then, continuing to do the same thing every day is NOT going to get you there. Makes sense, right? So, then it also makes sense that you've got to figure out a new approach...or as Einstein would suggest a new way of thinking! That's why I wrote this book...to give you a new way of looking at things, a guide to help you change your life and a resource to answer your health, fitness and wellness questions.

But let's get back to Eden where Adam was the first Healthy Dude. What was it like for him there? He was fit, ate well, spent lots of time with his family (Eve) and had little if any stress in his life (well until that whole snake and apple incident at any rate). Now, bear with me for this next part...I did this in **Healthy Tart** and now it's the Dudes' turn. While we can't really recreate Eden...there is a concept of an easier, simpler, healthier life that I want you to visualize. VISUALIZE!?! Yes, I said bear with me, okay?

I know, besides likely thinking I'm a bit crazy for asking you to 'visualize' something, you're probably also thinking...Eden, forget Eden. You just want to make it through the day and whatever it takes to do that is what you'll do. I get it. I'm betting your real world is probably a bit more like this:

The alarm wakes you from a dead sleep but you're still exhausted because you struggled to fall asleep - again! You manage to get out of bed and stumble around the room as you slowly come to life. Now, you're running late so you hurry to get ready to start your day. You have to meet the carpool gang or catch the bus or hit the road in your own car...that you have to fill with gas that costs more per gallon every month! Breakfast is nothing more than an overpriced cup of coffee from a drive-thru espresso stand... who has time for more than that? And then you're off to fight your way to the office...drop off the dry cleaning...get the kids to school or whatever your morning is filled with before your day really begins

You listen to the radio in the car and there's another burn ban issued because air pollution levels are too high. As you hear this, you notice almost every car, truck and bus on the road is spewing ugly exhaust into an already questionable air.

Traffic makes you late to the office or your first appointment, and you know you've got a project due by the end of the day...that you're behind on finishing...the day already seems out of control. You log onto your computer to find an onslaught of emails that you just don't have time to answer...spend the morning wading through your inbox and trying to reach the people you need to connect with in order to meet your project deadline. By late afternoon and after at least a pot of coffee, you realize you haven't eaten...but who has time to stop now?

So, it's the office vending machine with choices A5 and C3...something salty, something sweet! And, that's good eating?? Finally it's time to head home...having worked late to finish your project, but traffic is still a mess because of countless construction projects.

By the time you pull into your driveway you barely have the energy to get out of the car. You're famished and manage to find something packaged and frozen to 'nuke' in the microwave. You grab a cold beer and sit on the sofa to sort through a stack of mail...including too many bills you need to pay ASAP. You manage to get a few checks written before you fall asleep on the sofa. A few hours later you wake up with a terrible crick in your neck and fight exhaustion to get up and fall into your bed. Of course, then you start thinking about tomorrow's to-do list and projects...which keeps you from falling back to sleep.

Any of that sound a bit too familiar? See...visualizing isn't too hard, is it? Now I want you to think about a life without so many distractions and challenges...fewer deadlines and more free time...a life where living and thriving is second nature. What might this "Eden" in the modern world look like?

You wake up feeling completely rested...and have the whole day in front of you, which you're ready to face with energy to spare. The weather is perfect...not too hot, not too cold...so you head outside. You find yourself walking at a very brisk pace, or maybe even jogging, because you're fit and strong. As you look up into the clear blue sky you see nothing...no haze, no smog, no pollution...just bright skies. You take a deep breath of that amazing fresh, clean air and it powers you on as you walk, jog, run or whatever. Then you take a big swig from a bottle of water you've brought with you...filled right from your own tap. And, you can refill it at any stream, river, fountain or faucet you find because all accessible water is naturally clean. There is no need for filters, pumps or sanitizers...all accessible water is just naturally clean.

When you get a little hungry you stop at a stand to get a tasty sandwich or wrap that you know has nothing but fresh, wholesome ingredients...no added colors, flavors or chemicals. Then you stop by the neighborhood park and join in a pick up game of basketball...thrilled that you've still got the speed and moves to outplay almost everyone on the court.

Later you swing by the local farmer's market to select from an abundance of fresh fruits, vegetables and breads for your dinner. Everything is grown locally and made naturally...and there's so much to choose from you can barely decide. But, you can sample anything and everything that looks good right on the spot. Because no one uses pesticides, you don't have worry...just take a bite!

When you get back home you decide to prepare all your fresh food to make an amazing meal...fresh vegetables, maybe a little fish. Nothing is pre-packaged, ready made or processed...just healthy, nutritious and good tasting dishes that you and all your family and friends can't wait to dive into and enjoy. Yes, that's a typical experience...everyone eating together, laughing and sharing the day's highlights.

Days like this, with a steady diet of nutritious foods, regular exercise and good company means you're always healthy. No stress, no illness, no allergies...just you living your best life...every day. Wouldn't that be great? If life were really like this, getting and staying healthy would be easy, right?

But, we've already established that your day has too much stress, too much to do and no time for yourself. And, of course, you know that working too many hours, not getting enough sleep and exercise and poor eating habits is no way to live. It keeps you from having the energy and stamina you deserve and it can even shorten your life! But don't worry – even if your world seems dangerously close to the hectic reality described above and miles from that idyllic Eden...there is hope! I promise you that you can take some serious steps towards a more Eden-like lifestyle.

Healthy Dude gives you the steps you need to simplify your life, create an eating and exercise plan that you can stick with and address every health issue you have from bad breath to your sex drive. Now understand that I realize you can't stop everything else in your life and do nothing but focus on your health for the next 30-days. You've still got to work, spend time with your family and friends and take care of a long list of responsibilities. And, there's no way you're going to give up some of our modern conveniences like cell phones, laptops and bottled water. But don't worry...I am not going to send you out to live in a tent with a lantern and a list of edible leaves. I've written Healthy Dude as a sane and doable way for you to claim your corner of Eden amid your crazy real world. And, while following this program won't actually help you meet work deadlines, it will give you more energy and focus so you can meet those deadlines faster and easier, with energy to spare...and that's a major accomplishment!

Now, here's where my approach differs from some of the many 'quick-fix' plans and programs you've seen on TV and read about in books. I'm not promising you success overnight – or even in 30 days. I am talking about lifestyle changes you'll be able to live with – and thrive on – forever. So, I encourage you to take on one change at a time until you feel comfortable with that one change before you take on another. That is unless there's a major health risk involved and drastic measures are needed. If that's the case, a visit to www.TrishaStewart.com is in order to get more personalized support for your health challenge.

So, why do I recommend you make one change at a time? Remember last January's list of New Year's resolutions? Those business goals you set to accomplish in 3 months? How are those things going? Right! You see when we try to change everything in our lives at the same time, it can be overwhelming and before you know it you've dropped all the changes and are right back where you started. The best way to make lifestyle changes is to settle into one before you take on another. That way your changes will be entrenched in your life like brushing your teeth. I want to set you up for success...not failure. That's why I've created the 9-step program, the 30-day detox, shopping lists, an exercise plan and more...to give you the tools you need to reach your health and fitness goals one step at a time.

And the great thing is that if you need more guidance on getting started, customizing your plan due to health challenges or sticking with it for the long-term...there's support, information and coaching available through my website. So, just log onto www.TrishaStewart.com and change your life...one step at a time.

Chapter 2

9 Steps to Being a Healthy Dude

"With a definite, step-by-step plan - ah, what a difference it makes! You cannot fail, because each step carries you along to the next, like a track..." Scott Reed

It all starts with the first step...like getting out of bed first thing in the morning, picking up the phone to make that call or throwing out that last pack of cigarettes. Whatever your goals and dreams are, your best chance for success is to break it all down into a series of steps that you can accomplish one at a time. Sometimes your dreams are big...and they should be! But, looking at all you need to do to make that dream come true can be overwhelming. That's why a plan of action, a series of steps, is so important.

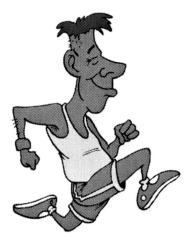

It helps you move ahead and allows you to look back every once in a while to see and remember how far you've already come...how much you've already done. You may realize that steps are needed for business and financial goals, but you might easily over look a 'plan' when it comes to health goals.

Well, this chapter is all about helping you create your plan of action and giving you step-by-step guidelines to reach your health and fitness goal.

So, you've decided you like the idea of a more Eden-like lifestyle, right? Whether it's having more energy, getting rid of the spare tire around your middle or you've got some major health concerns you'd like to address (and reverse!)...you're ready to live a better, healthier, happier life! Congratulations! You're well on your way to Healthy Dudedom...okay I made that word up, but you know what I mean. And, now you're thinking, how do I get started? What do I do? Can I even do this?

First, yes you can do this! You need to focus in on your personal goal...what is it that you want to accomplish and why. The WHY is what's going to keep you going when it gets hard, when you stumble or fall, or when you're tired and would rather lounge on the sofa and eat pizza? So, what's your WHY? Here's a few to think about:

- o   Adding quality years to your life (no nursing home for you!)
- o   Being able to compete in a marathon, finish a bike race or scale a mountain
- o   Keeping up with your kids
- o   Being around when your kids grow up
- o   Looking good for your class reunion, wedding or other special occasion
- o   Enjoying life rather than surviving it
- o   Curing a disease or major health challenge

One of these may light a spark inside you, or it may be something else. The only thing that matters is that you have your WHY...the reason you want to do this...and it's a reason that's important to you. It doesn't matter how badly someone else wants you to be healthy, you have to want it for yourself. Okay, you've got your WHY - now how do you get started?

No matter what your goals are, it all starts at the beginning. I've created Nine Steps to Being a Healthy Dude so that you can easily, systematically reach your goals. These steps cover the basics - inside and out - to being a healthy dude. A couple of them are so important (Eating and Exercise) that I've got follow up chapters to go into more detail. The others...we'll get into right here in this chapter. If you've got some specific concerns or are looking for some alternative answers...I talk about all of that in upcoming chapters. I know you might want to skip ahead and read what I have to say about your libido, whether acupuncture is right for you, or what you can do about your depression. That's fine...because that issue is probably connected to your WHY. But, please come back and read about the steps...because I want you to be a total Healthy Dude.

Here's a quick peek at the Nine Steps to Being a Healthy Dude:

1. Get Your Head on Straight *(Attitude affects your Health AND the Aging Process)*
2. Get your ZZZZZ's *(Sleeping lets you Re-Create yourself nightly)*
3. Stop Freaking Out *(Diffusing and Avoiding Stress)*

4. Have Good Hair Days *(Healthy hair and beard care)*

5. You don't have to be metro-sexual but...*(Nails, Skin & Smelling Good)*

6. A dirty mouth is out *(oral hygiene and fresh breath)*

7. Dress the part *(Clothes Really Do Make the Man)*

8. Eat to live well *(Healthy Dude Eating 101)*

9. Build Sweat Equity *(Exercise Increases Your Body's Value)*

Let's get started with, of course, Step One!

Step One: Get Your Head On Straight
(Attitude affects your Health AND the Aging Process)

"How young can you die of old age?" Stephen Wright

Men are living longer. (I know, this step is about attitude but bear with me, this relates to getting your head straight - I promise.) They say 65 is the new middle age (it used to be 50). And, most of you in your 40s and 50s will likely live to be more than 100 years old! So, I guess that means 40 is the new 30, which means 30 is the new 20...so 20 is the new 10? Okay...forget that...you 20 year-olds are still adults! It just means you've got decades more active years ahead of you than previous generations. But, only if you do it right. You see, these days many older men are not in the best of health...they're living lives full of prescribed medication, artificial hips and inactivity. I don't want you great, amazing men reading this book to be like that.

Think about this: In generations past, it was uncommon for men to live past the age of 50; then 50 became middle age and now 50 means you're just getting started. That's all great news, but hitting the 50 mark can still be a challenge if you don't take care of yourself. Men who have abused their bodies with junk food, alcohol and smoking, or are recovering from heart attacks and strokes – to them 50 still feels like 80 and every day can be a struggle. The bottom line: Don't become blasé about your health! You know that, right? I mean it's probably one of the reasons you're reading this book.

Now, realize that not being 'old' doesn't mean you won't have some signs of aging. Those little grey flecks in your sideburns, beard or through your hairline can happen at any age from the early twenties onwards. A few laughter or frown lines usually give men a bit of distinguished character. But you can feel younger and reduce or eliminate many of the visible signs of aging by avoiding too much sun, stress, poor diet and smoking...these make you old before your time! And, I'm going to address those things in some later steps. But, before you restock your refrigerator, create an exercise plan or get your look updated...you've GOT to GET YOUR HEAD ON STRAIGHT! You've got to have the right attitude about being healthy.

Maybe you've heard it before...attitude is everything. Okay, it takes more than positive thoughts to get in shape (at some point you have to lift a weight, swim a lap or put down the pizza), but a positive mental attitude will keep you focused and on track. Stop thinking about what's wrong with you; where you fall short; what you wish you looked like. You are where you are...start from there and move forward. Picture how you'd look at your peak of physical fitness and good health...keep that image in your mind and know that's where you're headed. If you focus on where you're going...you'll just keeping moving...and that positive attitude supports your zest for life, your joy in moving and exercising, and your pleasure in eating well. And...are you ready for this...it keeps you feeling and looking younger. And, can actually slow and reverse the aging process! Seriously...just adding a smile can take years off your face. Imagine if you didn't just smile, but actually felt happy and positive on the inside as well. Hmmmm...

Now, let me clear up what I mean by positive attitude. I don't mean you have to be one of those people who always see the good in everything. Let's be honest, those 'perpetually sunny, never a cloud in the sky' people can be just a bit annoying – don't you think? What I mean by having a positive attitude that will improve your health and slow your aging is that you look to the future. You have a plan in place and are excited about it. Now your big plan may be about your career, your retirement, your passion...but we're going to focus on the health aspect of your plan. Because, no matter what you envision yourself doing in 5 years...10 years...20 years...if you're not healthy, you won't be doing it. So...plug your health and fitness goals into your plan.

There are a few different things you can do to keep the right mental attitude and to think and feel young. First, there's mental stimulation! For most of us, once we got out of school that was the end of daily mental exercise. So, if it's been a while since you challenged yourself mentally – take it easy. I don't want you to strain your brain! Seriously, any form of learning and challenging yourself mentally keeps you alert and keeps your brain stimulated. So, skip stagnant and go straight to supercharged! From reading books to taking classes to doing crossword puzzles, keep those synapses firing!

You can also hang out with people younger than you...no matter your age...and that will keep you acting younger and moving more. Okay, you may need longer rest periods than your younger buddies, but it really does help. Nothing is quite so challenging as being told you're the 'old guy' on the team, right? As long as you don't overdo it in trying to prove yourself, it can be just the motivation you need. So hit the local park or gym for a game of basketball, sign up for your company's softball team or just join a club. Get involved and stay active so you can get fit and stay young.

That's the best solution because so far, there is no fountain of youth. Yes, scientists are working on some sort of potion or pill...but wouldn't it be better to stay young naturally? I think so. Of course, you are going to age...every year you get older...that's the way you're made. But, why is it some men age faster than others...some 70 year olds look 50 and some 50 year olds look 80? It's about the choices you make. The great thing is that it doesn't matter where you are and how you feel right now...you're going to get better, feel stronger, younger and fitter...and be happier...if you start to live your life the Healthy Dude way.

Step Two - Get your ZZZZZ's
(Sleeping lets you Re-Create yourself nightly)

"No matter what time it is, wake me, even if it's in the middle of a Cabinet meeting." Ronald Reagan

---

Seems everybody has an idea about sleep...how to do it, what mattress is best, how much you need and what to do if you're not getting enough. Clearly it's an important part of your daily activity. In fact, I prefer to call sleeping *re-creation*...it's a time when we rest and recuperate our body and mind (hopefully) and ready ourselves to start a new day with lots of energy and motivation. Sounds nice, doesn't it? But that's not always the case. Overworked, overtired, overfed, overstressed...there are a lot of factors that keep you from getting enough sleep. Even when you work can do a number on your nightly nap!

Typically you hear that everyone needs eight hours of sleep each night, but that actually varies from person to person. Some people are at the top of their game with only six hours, while others feel better when they get nine. And, just so you understand that 'normal' is a relative term, check this out...giraffe's only sleep 1.5 hours a day, while a python sleeps about 18! But, no matter what your 'optimum number of sleep hours', actually getting that quality sleep is the real challenge. There are those of you who would love to sleep more if

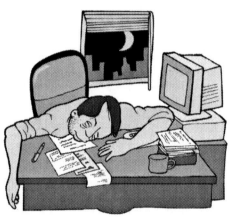

schedule allowed and some who have the time but just can't get to sleep...or fall asleep only to wake up a short time later. The right kind of restorative (re-creating) sleep is far too elusive for many of you. So, how can you fix it?

Certainly there are sleep disorders that can affect your rest...and I'll get to some of those in a bit. But, for many of you, how you sleep is really a habit...and that habit can be good or bad. For example, if you always go to bed at midnight but can't get up in the morning when the alarm goes off at 6am...you need to go to bed earlier. Despite the fact you don't feel tired until midnight – your body needs more than those six hours. Besides, going to bed at midnight is just a habit...so change it and create a new habit of going to bed earlier. Another example is the man who goes to bed early at say 9:30pm, but can't actually GET to sleep until around 3am. He's got the habit of going to bed at a certain time but his body doesn't need that much sleep... so he needs to wait to go to bed until he's actually tired. And for those who fall asleep only to wake up a few hours later; that can be signs of stress, what's in your room or what you're doing right before bed.

If you're one of those who have trouble with sleep...there are also some things that you should remove from your bedroom: Televisions, computers, phones, PDAs and other electronic gadgets. Believe it or not, the energy from these things actually disturbs sleep patterns - even the electronic clock! I'm sure you're thinking – Trisha, I have to have my clock. Well, if you have trouble getting enough restful sleep - move it to another part of the room and set the alarm to wake you.

Think about it - you really don't need to know what time it is if you wake in the night. And, as far as what you're doing before bed...don't eat a huge meal (ideally eat no later than 7pm and take a quick stroll if possible). If you do end up eating late...keep it simple and avoid animal protein and high energy carbohydrates. Also, remember that alcohol and coffee are stimulants... and while a glass of red wine has some benefits, drinking the entire bottle will dehydrate you and keep you up. I like the idea of the Chinese Clock. It divides up the entire day with peak hours for each part of your body (organs). Take a look at the diagram... notice when each body part is at its peak activity. This is very helpful in figuring out, for example, when to eat.

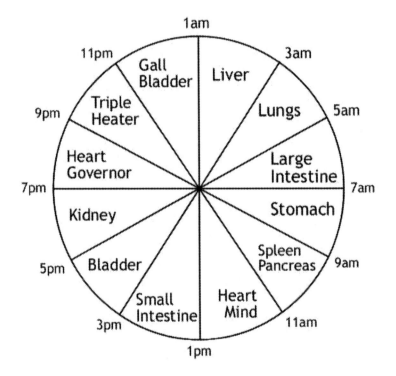

Let's look at the liver, with 'peak activity' hours from 1-3am. You want to be done eating long enough before those peak hours (say 6 or 7pm as suggested above) so that the liver can really do its part in the digestive process by 1am. Makes sense, right? Because if you're busy eating at midnight, your liver can't work on that food for almost 25 hours! Whew...no wonder you can't sleep after that late night snack....it's just sitting there in your gut!

The strongest time for our liver is between 1 - 3am, we should be sleeping soundly, our digestive system should be rested, allowing the blood to be pooled back to regenerate ready for another day of full and exciting activities.

By eating too late or not sleeping properly, the blood is unable to be stored back into the liver and therefore cannot be regenerated properly. Look at it as if you are charging your mobile phone - if you use the in-car charger too often you will deplete the battery quicker because it is charging too quickly. If you plug it in overnight, the battery lasts longer.......

You may be thinking, "Okay it'd be great if I got more – or at least better – sleep. But, what's the harm really?" You get through the day, get most of the things done on your to-do list and you might even say "I've got too much to do...I can sleep when I'm dead!" Well, hold up there dude! What exactly happens to you if you don't get the adequate sleep your body needs? First it's little things you notice, like struggling to pay attention in that afternoon meeting, forgetting a few little things like returning that phone call or picking up the dry cleaning (or the kids from soccer practice)! And it gets worse from there...your response time goes up, your effectiveness goes down. Bottom line...you think you're getting more done with less sleep, but really you're not doing any of it as well as you can.

Sometimes though, your sleep troubles are more severe than needing to have one less beer, moving the TV and changing your bed time. There are, in fact, several sleep disorders that can really disrupt your natural sleep cycle. Let's take a look at the main troublemakers: insomnia, sleep apnoea, Restless Leg Syndrome (RLS) and narcolepsy.

Insomnia

The most general description of insomnia is difficulty or inability to fall asleep (whether you're tired or not). Other symptoms or versions of insomnia include:

- o Being unable to sleep unless taking alcohol or sleeping pills
- o Lying awake at night unable to sleep
- o Waking up in the middle of the night and unable to go back to sleep
- o Awakening in the morning too early despite being tired and feeling un-refreshed
- o Falling asleep in the day, needing to nap, feeling drowsy and lacking concentration

Insomnia happens to many people during their life and is often a short term challenge due to stress, differing time zones when travelling and changes in diet or medication. However, insomnia can also be long term due to extreme unhappiness, some types of prescribed medications and poor bedtime habits. While insomnia is never a good thing, long-term insomnia should be treated.

Certainly, relaxation CDs at bedtime with the headphones can be of great help, as can herbal preparations. For more personalized help and/or support, register on my website at www.trishastewart.com. (Also, see chapter 7 for further information).

Sleep Apnoea

Sleep apnoea is a very traumatic, life threatening problem. The scary thing is that many sufferers don't know they have the problem until their bed partner hears them choking and gasping for breath. Or worse, they sometimes stop breathing for a few seconds! What's going on when that happens is a restriction in the respiratory airways that causes the deprivation of oxygen. While obstructive sleep apnoea sufferers often snore, this is not the same as normal snoring. And, there's also CSA - Central Sleep Apnoea - that does not cause snoring. Our brain signal's us to breathe, but CSA suffers have a delay in that signal, which causes the body to stop breathing. This can be caused by a stroke, brain tumor, viral brain disease or a chronic respiratory problem. If you suffer from sleep apnoea, it's important that you get it treated...start working with the 30 day plan as diet will help but also talk to your doctor.

Restless Leg Syndrome (RLS)

RLS typically occurs when you try to rest, which means it can occur in the daytime. Have you ever been so tired that your body actually twitches? You're lying in bed and you have the uncontrollable feeling to move your legs...they feel hot and are twitching. That's RLS! And, it makes sleep very elusive and difficult. There are treatments for RLS that include natural supplements such as magnesium, changing in bed habits, and relaxation techniques.

Narcolepsy

You've probably seen narcolepsy used as a joke in some film or TV show...someone falls asleep in the middle of a sentence or activity. Seems funny, but it's actually quite dangerous because the sufferer can truly fall asleep anywhere without notice...driving, walking, working, on the phone, during face to face conversations...literally anything. Narcolepsy is a neurological disorder where the brain cannot differentiate between when to be asleep and when to be awake. The sufferer can experience extreme wakefulness, heart palpitations, hallucinations, being asleep while doing something and then having no memory of it. Believe it or not, narcolepsy can happen to any of us at some time because the biggest cause is extreme stress – and we can all have too much stress in our lives. For anyone who feels they may have narcolepsy, it's important to understand you may need treatment. For further information, see chapter 7 or go to my website at www.trishastewart.com.

Sleep – true quality, restorative sleep is a vital part of being a Healthy Dude. If you want to learn a bit more about what's actually going on while you sleep (Non-REM and REM stages), then checkout my website at www.trishastewart.com. But, if you are suffering from any sleep disorders, or think you may be, you should seek treatment. I believe the majority, if not all, sleep issues can be addressed and corrected through the right diet, exercise and sleep habits. If you need more advice on getting better sleep or treating a sleep disorder, visit my website – www.TrishaStewart.com and I'll answer your questions and provide the support you need to ensure a good night's rest!

Step Three - Stop Freaking Out
(Diffusing and Avoiding Stress)

"Brain cells create ideas. Stress kills brain cells. Stress is not a good idea." Frederick Saunders

Well, you just read how stress can affect your sleep...but let's look more closely at stress...what it is...how it affects your health...and what you can do about it. So, what exactly is stress? You hear the word on a daily basis, but what is it? Simply put, it's the inability to adapt to change. That 'change' is something, anything, that causes you to feel uneasy, unsure or anxious - pressure from work, bosses and colleagues, finances, family, society, religion, politics, racial issues and more!

Okay, so stress is out there – we have deadlines, bills to pay, obligations to meet, goals to reach, decisions to make – but how and why does it affect our health and well-being? It starts with changing or altering our emotions, but ongoing stress actually changes our physiology. Many of my clients have heard me say, "Mind invades body." In other words, we feel the pressure, it makes us anxious and the next thing you know we can't eat because our stomach's upset or we get a

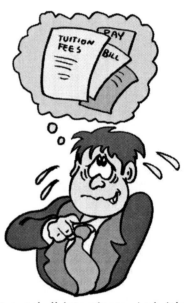

headache that threatens to split our skull into pieces. And, it's not just adults. Do you ever remember feeling nervous as a child? Maybe that first time you had to get up in front of the class and give a report? First, you were worried you wouldn't do a good job, then you got those "butterflies" in your stomach making you feel a little 'sick to your stomach', and before you knew it you were tossing your cookies in the hallway (if you made it that far). Okay - that wasn't you, I know, it was that other kid...but you remember it, right? So, why does that happen? Well, it all comes from a direct hormone response... sending a signal to the brain, which sends the signal to the vagus nerve (attached to the brain stem), that signal travels down to the esophagus and into the stomach. So, from nerves to nausea...just like that!

If mild stress can make you throw up (or want to), imagine what severe or prolonged stress can do. Enough stress and your health can be seriously compromised: weakened immune system, fatigue, high blood pressure, diabetes, heart attack, headaches, and stomach disorders including ulcers, asthma - even eczema - all due to stress! So, the simple thing to do is get rid of stress, right? Well, unfortunately you really can't. Stress is outside forces that insist on those changes – remember? But, what you can change is how you deal with stress and ways to lessen its effects on you and your body. I'm sure you know what I'm going to say – but the ability to handle and respond to stress is increased by a good diet, enough exercise and adequate rest and relaxation. Believe me...these three things are the key to having balance in your life and being a Healthy Dude.

Now I'm going to specifically talk about eating and exercise as separate steps, but before we get to that...I want to share some things that will help you combat stress in your life.

1. **Have a good belly laugh!** Really, when was the last time you actually felt your belly shaking because of laughter (instead of just shaking because you've got a bit too much fat around the middle)? Laughing produces those happy hormones we call endorphins, which help you to relax. So rent a silly movie, watch a comedian or just call a friend who tells good jokes. Laughter really is good medicine. In fact, anything that releases those endorphins...exercise, excitement and orgasm...help relieve stress. The next time you experience any of these - notice that morphine-like effect on the body that just makes you want to lay back and relax afterwards...fantastic stress busters!

2. **Seven-Eleven Breathing!** Here's a quick way to de-stress I learned from a colleague who specializes in helping people deal with stress. You breathe in to the count of seven and breathe out to the count of 11. Do this six times and you will truly feel better. Remember this technique the next time you're stuck in traffic, can't fix a problem, or just need time to think about what you are going to do about a situation.

3. **Learn to meditate!** No, this is not just for monks...you can use meditation daily to release all your negative thoughts so that new and positive ones can come replace them. If meditation is new to you...just try something that allows you to slow down and not focus on all the thoughts racing through

your head. Just 10 minutes of stretching or yoga can really help regenerate your mind and body. Take a nice warm bath or massage your scalp in the shower. Better still get your partner to give you an Indian head massage...which is described in Chapter 7 if you're not familiar.

4. Take a vacation! Make sure you plan vacations and breaks into your schedule. One two-week vacation a year is not enough. Add a few weekend getaways or day trips that are just for fun. That means get out of the office, get away from home and leave the phones, computers and gadgets behind... YES, and turn that cell phone off.

All this stress can cause havoc on your body - the liver, kidneys, lungs and all the associated systems and organs are under pressure and fighting for survival. So, clearly it makes sense to not only find ways to handle stress, but to reduce or avoid stressful situations when possible. You need to find out what exactly causes you to feel uncomfortable and find a way of making some changes. There may be some changes you can make from working different hours and saying "no" to more commitments to getting needed moral support and ending toxic relationships. But remember it's not always possible to eliminate the cause of your stress and no one's life is completely stress free. But, there is always a way of working around it and through it. In Chapter Seven I talk about some alternative techniques and therapies that might be the answer you've been looking for to combat your stressful life.

Step Four - Have Good Hair Days
(Healthy hair and beard care)

"Gray hair is God's graffiti" Bill Cosby

I know this is going to shock you, but the health of your hair is

very dependent on your diet! I know, here I go again saying the right diet is the answer, but it is so true. So, why am I talking about your hair as a part of being a Healthy Dude? Because, the outer you needs to be just as healthy as the inner you if you want to be a completely Healthy Dude. And, who doesn't want to look good, right?

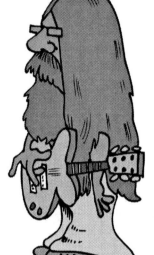

Let's start with the basics. I know it seems obvious that you should wash your hair, but I have to ask... what are you washing it with? Men don't always want to bother with special shampoos and conditioners, but you need to. Trust me, that body shampoo is not multi-purpose. So, don't believe that if it's good enough for your body, it's good enough for your hair. It ain't so. First of all, it's likely to be full of chemicals like lauryl sulphates and other nasty things. These will dry the skin on your scalp and cause the white dust you find on your dark clothing or that awful stuff that looks like rock salt falling out of your hair onto everything including the car seats. YUK!

Cheap products don't help you in the long run. You need a good quality, gentle product made of natural ingredients and essential oils. There are plenty on the market, but read the labels. Just because something says it has natural scents or oils doesn't mean it doesn't contain chemicals.

So, your hair is clean, but maybe it's turning grey. Don't panic...luckily most men get that 'distinguished' look when those grey temples start to appear. If you can't handle that, you can get your hair colored - again there are natural products out there. The most important thing is to be sure you've got a good hairstylist cutting your hair on a regular basis. He or she can give you specific advice about your hair care needs. And, if you have a mustache or beard - please keep it clean, neat and trimmed. If you don't like to do it yourself...have your stylist keep you clipped. A neat goatee or nice moustache can be quite dashing and sexy, but on the other hand - nothing is as unappealing on a man's face as scruffy, dirty, shaggy facial hair.

Now, let's talk about it...the lack of hair. Most men deal with hair loss at some point in their life...some much younger than others. But it all comes down to how you deal with it. It may be male pattern baldness, but before you right it off as inevitable, realize that some hair loss is a result of stress or trauma. There are treatments for that. Yes, some of those hair loss pills and potions can help, but first try some good vitamins – a B complex, C, E and Selenium can help, and be sure you're getting enough Omega 3', 6', 9's in your diet or from supplements. There are several ways to deal with hair loss from getting a hair piece or hair transplant (they've come a long way with both) or just shaving your head and going for the bald look. It works for many stars and athletes...and can be quite attractive. However, please, please do NOT under ANY circumstances comb your hair over to cover a bald spot. You're not fooling anyone and it actually makes you look older, not younger. So DON'T DO IT!!!

Step Five - Be metro-sexual...sort of
(The Importance of nails, skin & smelling good)

Beauty is only skin deep, but *it's a* valuable asset *if you're poor or haven't any sense.* **Vernon Howard**

Don't panic! I'm not going to tell you to that you have to get a weekly manicure or take hour long mud baths...but for the entire Healthy Dude package, you've got to pay attention to your skin and nails. So, while you might not become metro-sexual, a little time and attention to your extremities will help you look completely pulled together and be sure that your skin and nails are able to do their job.

Strong nails are great actually tools we need....they help us scratch things, peel fruit, open things, pick away the outer layers of edibles, undo knots and perform a 'boat-load' of other great things. And, your skin...well first it's the largest organ of your body...plus it serves as the protector for everything inside...from veins to joints to organs. So, let's take a closer look at nails and skin.

Don't think your fingernails are very useful? Seriously do you really never have to untie a knot or open the pull tab of a cold beverage? Here's a little experiment...cut your nails down to the quick and bandage or tape them up...then see how you do for a day. Okay, you don't really have to do that...but if you need some convincing, give it a try. Just don't cut the nail too short or it can become ingrown – and that's NO FUN. Enough of that...we've established that you need your fingernails (and toenails too for that matter)!

Now...how do you care for them? For men, ideally, you don't really notice the nails when they're neatly trimmed, clean and healthy. But if a man has dirty fingernails (often from work I understand), it can be the only thing people notice. Want to hold hands with your date? Forget it! You don't have to spend a lot of time...and you can probably keep your nails looking good all by yourself. But, if you've never had a manicure...give it a shot. The deep soaking, softening and cleaning up the cuticles (that skin that has grown up over the base of your nail) is often best left to the experts. Then they can clean, cut and buff your nails to a nice healthy shine.

No – you do NOT have to put on clear nail polish...I promise. And, here's a quick trick for manicure health...after every shower or bath as you're drying off...take your towel and use it to push back your cuticles. Your cuticles are softened because of the water and the towel is a safe way to push back cuticles with no risk of cutting or injuring yourself.

Same goes for your feet! Speaking of feet, if your toenails get too long...your shoes won't fit right and you'll feel pain...not a good thing. So simply keeping all your nails clean and trimmed is huge. And it won't hurt to slap a little lotion on your hands and feet...this keeps your cuticles soft. Don't think it matters? Well, then you've never had a cuticle get too dry and crack...bleed and cause serious discomfort? And, if it's never happened, you don't want it to!

Toe Tips
- Use a foot file and file off any hard skin on the heels and around the big toes
- Put some baking soda and skin or bath oil into a bowl of warm water and soak your feet, using an old toothbrush brush the sides of the toenails where all those bits of sock get stuck.
- If there is any chance you have a problem with athlete's foot, get some Citricidal or tea tree oil and clean up

daily. This will help to prevent and clear up any fungal infection. If the toe nails are yellow you have a severe fungal infection, check for other signs such as "jock itch" this is another tell tale sign of fungal infection. Check into www.trishastewart.com for further advice.

- Trim the toenails with proper nail clippers, do not cut down too far into the corner as you will risk getting an ingrown toenail which is very painful
- Get some moisture cream and slap it on those lovely clean feet
- Finally, push back the cuticles with a cuticle stick or pen.

Let's move on to your skin. Did you know that you have about 5 – 6.5 feet of skin covering your body? That's a lot of skin...but then it has a big job. Primarily, it protects your body from injury and infection (or the invasion of microbes). Imagine how careful you'd have to be if you walked around with your muscles and veins and organs exposed! Along with covering your insides, your skin contains sensory nerve endings that are sensitive to touch, temperature, pressure and pain...sending messages to pull your hand back from that hot stove or put on a jacket when it's cold. Besides altering you to temperature changes, your skin actually helps your hormonal system regulate your body temperature, plus it's one of the excretory organs together with the lungs, kidneys and bowel. In other words it helps get rid of toxins and waste in your body – primarily through sweating, which I'll get back to in a bit.

Needless to say, the skin has a huge job to do...and for the most part you ignore it, abuse it and brutalize it. Seriously, how often do you 'think' about your skin? You get it dirty, scrape it up, bang it around, scratch it and bruise it. And, beyond getting a daily wash (often with a harsh, drying soap) you take it for granted. Certainly there are some of you who are more aware of your skin; you may even have a skin condition like eczema or psoriasis (which I talk about in more detail in Chapter 5). But, the majority of you reading this book need to give a little more thought to skin care...where would you be without it?

Here's the cool thing – it's much more acceptable in today's society for men to pay attention to personal grooming and skin care. There are even many wonderful salon treatments just for men. And, about that harsh, old school soap you're using? Please, buy something else...go for natural, chemical free products. It's better for your skin and besides, you already take in enough chemicals and pollutants through the environment...no need to add to it with your cleansing products.

Speaking of products...let's talk a little about sweating (I told you I'd come back to that). Since sweating is a healing, detoxifying process for your body, you don't want to eliminate it. Yet, who doesn't slather on the deodorant every morning before you hit the road? Sure, you want to smell nice, but guess what...most of the odor from your sweat has to do with your diet! There I go again, stressing the importance of what you're eating. But, it's true...if you have a healthy diet - your sweat won't have the offensive odors you're concerned about. I realize you might not believe me and if you're going out on a date you're likely not to take any chances. So, at least start using a more natural deodorant instead of one chock full of chemicals!

Have you ever really pampered yourself? If not, I encourage you to try a salon/spa treatment. Come on, you can try it at least once! Get a facial, a mud wrap, a paraffin wax for your hands...the works. Maybe you're not ready to try it all...but give one of them a shot and I bet you'll love it. Then, think about going in for a monthly treatment. You'll feel relaxed, calm and healthy - plus it does wonders for your confidence. And, while you're in the spa, have them take a look at your unwanted body hair. Not every man struggles with this, but for those that do it can be a real problem and if it bothers you - lose it! From 'mono-brow' to shaggy back hair...there are ways to get rid of it. There are professional procedures like a wax treatment (WARNING: VERY PAINFUL) or the more permanent solution of laser therapy. Please be sure you leave these procedures to experts, not someone who just learned how to heat up the wax! You can also try shaving your back and chest (body builders often do this). While it's a treatment you can do at home - you may need help with your back. And, please be careful of ingrown hair. A great way to reduce that problem is to use a body brush and exfoliate your skin on a regular basis. You can buy the products you need at most bath shops - again keep the products natural if possible.

Remember, I'm not saying you have to spend hours in the spa or bathroom, but adding a bit more grooming time to your nails and skin helps you look like the healthy dude you're becoming on the inside!

Step Six - A dirty mouth is out
(Oral hygiene and fresh breath)

"I told my dentist my teeth are going yellow... he told me to wear a brown tie." Rodney Dangerfield

---

Speaking of the inside...it's time to talk about your breath! Did you know that bad breath is not necessarily caused by your teeth or gums? Sometimes, oftentimes, it's a result of something much further down in the digestive system. But, since you're going to be working on getting a healthier diet, that type of bad breath shouldn't be a problem. So, for this step, I want to concentrate on your oral cavity.

The oral cavity is made up of your teeth, gums, tongue and salivary glands. They all do their part to help you taste, enjoy and digest food. But it's what's left behind after that great meal that can cause the problems. All the food and bacteria in your mouth can build up along your gum line and around your teeth...this is what we call plaque. When it hardens it becomes tartar. It's something we all have to deal with, although some of us build up plaque and tarter more quickly than others. And it's all that plaque and bacteria that give you smelly breath!

Luckily, it's easy to deal with. Brushing your teeth - and more importantly flossing - are the tools to fresh breath. Yes, you've heard your dentist harp on about flossing and while he may not be concerned about the social aspect of you having bad breath, he knows that's the beginning to real tooth decay and dental issues – even oral cancers. Remember, healthy teeth and gums are very sexy - the opposite is so NOT sexy or appealing on any level.

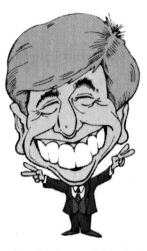

When you're selecting your toothpaste or mouthwash, please do not get one with added fluoride (you really don't need it) and other chemicals that should be nowhere near your mouth. There are lots of natural, 'free from' products to use. Even baking soda or a good sea salt are great alternatives. Sure, they don't foam up like what you're used to...but you'll have clean teeth and fresh breath naturally! Here's a tip – if you rush from meeting to meeting all day where you drink or eat, you may need a quick cleaning between appointments. Carry a small travel toothbrush or even handier one of those small dental-brushes you slip on your finger. It's a way to maintain that you're fresh all day long!

Step Seven - Dress the part
(Clothes Really Do Make the Man)

"Clothes make the man. Naked people have little or no influence on society." Mark Twain

---

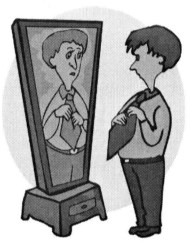

While men certainly have an easier time keeping up with fashion than women (seems women's styles change every 5 minutes), it's important to keep up to date. There are always the classic looks you can rely on, but certain looks are gone, baby, gone. Unless you're Hugh Hefner – lose the pipe, smoking jacket and slippers. And cardigans are best left to the golf course these days (and they've become a rare sighting even on the links). But, even if you're not a fashion plate, 'dressing to the nines' as it were, you still need to look pulled together, whatever your style.

A lot of how you dress depends on the job you do, since you spend more hours working each day than anything else. But whether you're a 'suit on Wall Street,' a tradesmen working in construction or somewhere in the middle, you need to wear quality, well cut clothes and shoes. Nothing is so sloppy looking as a suit jacket that pulls across the shoulders because it's too small or a pair of trousers hanging in all the wrong places. And please, if ANY of you out there are still wearing the super baggy, oversized jeans that are barely hanging on your hips so your boxers can show...STOP IT! Seriously, that look doesn't work for anyone and no matter what kind of shape you're in or how healthy you are...nobody's going to care.

Now some of you may have certain clothes you have to wear for work – uniforms or required clothing – but you can still control the fit of those clothes. And, when you're off the clock – show your style...flaunt your stuff!

If you are at a loss when it comes to picking out the right clothes for you – from fit, to style to color – then get some help. Shop at stores with employees who know their stuff! Then make their day by asking for some assistance. They will help you pull together the look that fits you, your style and your budget. Dressing well doesn't have to cost an arm and a leg – so don't worry if you're on a budget. Sure, it'll take an investment of time on your part to find the right wardrobe, but once you've got your closet set – you can pull out anything and know you'll look amazing! That's a great confidence boost – and that's the way Healthy Dudes do it!

Trisha Stewart

Step Eight - Eat to live Well

(Healthy Dude Eating 101)

"He who does not mind his belly, will hardly mind anything else." Samuel Johnson

Okay, you've heard me say in pretty much every step so far, how eating right is vital to your health. Well, now it's time to get into it a bit more. However, it's so important to me and to you becoming a Healthy Dude that the entire next chapter is devoted to giving you great information on how to eat...including the famous 30-day plan that works a dream on your waistline and energy levels!

Eating right really is the key to being healthy, because without this step you cannot fully function at your peak performance level. There are a number of conditions that can be caused by poor eating and treated – with great success – by healthy eating. Mood swings (even depression), migraine headaches, digestive disturbances, eczema, asthma, Type II diabetes and, of course, excess weight are all tightly linked to what you eat. You've heard 'garbage in, garbage out'...it's true.

So, what should you be eating and how much? Here's a quick lesson – if you're eating it in its original form (i.e., vegetables, fruit, nuts, grains) – it's good for you. If it comes in a package and has a long list of ingredients you can't pronounce – it's bad for you. I realize that's an over simplification and there are some gray areas involved, but it's a quick rule of thumb to keep in mind. I have to tell you that I am a vegetarian and I promote a healthy, balanced vegetarian diet. However, I am not going to tell you that you absolutely MUST eat like I do. Why? Because even though I believe it's the best way to eat, I know it's not a fit for everyone. In fact, I am sure a lot of you men would toss this book in the garbage if I said you could never grill another steak. However, I am going to give you some facts on meat so you can make informed, wise decisions. And, I'm going to share with you how to increase the amounts of good for you fruits, vegetables, grains, lentils, nuts and more into your diet without sacrificing taste – or the joy of eating. Fair enough? Great

Now would be a good time to take a look in your refrigerator, freezer and cupboards and do some serious cleaning. Toss out the stuff you don't recognize, that's covered with freezer burn and that's so packaged and preserved it won't go bad for another 20 years! You're going to fill up your house with fresh, natural foods which will sustain your body, keep you filled with energy and free of most of the health concerns you currently have. Don't worry, I provide a shopping list to get your started and lay out every step of my 30-day detox program to kick-start your way to becoming a Healthy Dude.

A big question for many of you is how much should you eat? How many calories do you really need every day? Well, portion size is out of control, so it's hard to judge what you should eat by how much you're served in any given restaurant. And, you need to factor in how active you are. If you sit at a desk all day, you'll need fewer calories than the professional athlete. It seems obvious, but most of you are eating far too many calories every day. We, by nature, overestimate how active we are and underestimate how much we eat. But the following chapters are going to help you reset your intake and output levels for food and exercise to get you on the right track.

9. Building Sweat Equity
(Exercise Increases Your Body's Value)

"Jogging is very beneficial. It's good for your legs and your feet. It's also very good for the ground. If makes it feel needed." Charles M. Schultz

---

Many years ago man did not take any exercise apart from his daily routine which was manual work. Look as far back as the first Dude - Adam - in Eden. As a hunter/gatherer he would have been out foraging for food all the time – no need for extra exercise then. These days too many men spend the day sitting...in a car, an office, in meetings, on the train, plane or bus...but sitting. Even those doing manual labor these days tend to only work a few limited muscles (mostly straining the lower back). But your bodies aren't meant for that limited motion, and really not for all that sitting around where you're folded into a position which is not natural. At least one-minute every hour you should be fully upright and stretched right out.

Go on, get out of the chair now and stretch up as tall as you can with your arms way above your head. Notice how your belly comes into your back and how all the muscles down the front of the body become longer and under the arms feels like it is going to stretch forever? What a great feeling...all the blood rushing around now instead of pushing through cramped up muscles. This will even make your digestive system work better. You can feel it all now moving – feet firmly on the ground stretching out the plantar fascia (bottoms of the feet), toes wriggling to keep you balanced...yes there are plenty of muscles, joints and connective tissues in those feet! I bet you can hear some creaking and groaning of joints that have not been in that position for way too long.

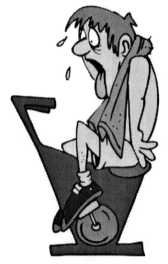

Should you be that stiff and tight? Well, watch a baby or youngster...their bodies are fluid. They can crouch down into a squat position and hold it for ages; they lie on their backs with legs completely "akimbo"; often you will see them asleep with their hands above their heads.

What happened to you? Well, you grew up (YUK!) and with becoming an adult came stress, working too hard and forgetting to actually keep practicing those things.

That's why exercise is so important these days. First, we're adults that forget to stretch and keep ourselves limber and flexible and second, we spend too much of our days (day after day) sitting and not moving and strengthening our bodies. So, you've got to increase the value of your body with some good exercise...get the heart pumping, the limbs moving and the muscles growing. Three things...that means three types of exercise:

Endurance: Aerobic exercise/cardiovascular that includes running, hiking, cycling, skiing anything that pushes the heart rate above its normal activity.

Strength: Muscle building/toning using primarily weight training and lifting heavy objects.

Flexibility: Keeping you limber with things like yoga, Pilates and simple stretching. Most men skip this and feel it's not important (or just for women), but you would feel so much better in every way if you stretched out more. Plus, it helps with balance, mental clarity, well being, depression, problem solving, and anxiety – all seems clearer when you have done a great routine.

The cool thing about exercise is that it not only makes your body feel better, but it improves your mood too...you'll just feel better, have more energy and get more done. All without the help of caffeine! Exercise increases cardio vascular fitness which means your heart muscles and circulatory system is strong, the lungs are pumping hard. Bottom line...the rest of the body has a greater chance of survival if your whole engine is roaring and pumping good blood, oxygen and nutrients around the body to feed the many cells and bring about good health. Your increased muscle strength will help with your posture, keep your bones in place and lessen your chances of low back, hip and knee pain. And, there are also hormonal system benefits with exercise (and yes, that can mean better sex!). You see, there is a release of endorphins – the "happy hormones" - which actually make us feel relaxed and happy.

Chapter 3

Healthy Dude Eating
Are you really what you eat?

One should eat to live, not live to eat. - **Benjamin Franklin**

Now there's a great thought, but one too often ignored. Don't believe me? Think about how you plan your day, your week and your social life...mostly around food. You have a business meeting: "Let's do lunch." You want to meet up with a good friend: "We'll meet for coffee, or a drink." You invite friends over to watch the game and if there aren't beer, nachos and pizza around, there will be trouble. Even dating: you have a first date over coffee, then its dinner, and drinks; Even going to the movies involves popcorn and sodas. And family...WOW...almost every family gathering is an exercise in over eating (and refusing food insults your Aunt Mildred who cooked for two days to feed you!). Certainly eating with friends and family is more fun than eating alone, but you need to be sure you're staying focused on only putting into

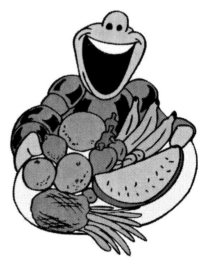

your mouth what your body needs. No, I'm not saying you can never have pizza again, but every weekend? What do you think? And, you may be asking, "Trisha, I work out enough, why does it matter what I actually eat?" Well...great question. *So, are you really what you eat?*

You've been hearing me for the previous two chapters (and in almost every step of the 9 steps) say how important eating right is for your overall health, vitality and well-being. So obviously, I would say that you are what you eat, right? Wrong...you are actually what you absorb. I know, it may sound like a minor technicality, but I'm going to explain a bit of how what you eat is actually used and you'll understand better. Then, I'll share with you some great information on nutrition, food groups and the best sources for the fats, proteins and carbohydrates you need. And, yes, I give you all the details you need for my famous 30-Day Detox!

It's really crazy how many different diet approaches and styles are out there...and most of them only lead to frustration and failure. So, it's no wonder whether you're overweight, underweight or even at your ideal weight that you probably aren't eating a healthy diet. But, with my years of experience as a nutritionist helping hundreds of clients, I truly believe I have the safe, real answers on what to eat, when to eat and the overall benefits and effects you should expect from your food. You'll learn about foods that affect your mood, your waistline and many common ailments. Trust me; my aim is not some quick-fix scheme to help you drop 10 pounds before next weekend. My goal is to give you the information and tools you need for long term change...so you can achieve your health goals and then maintain them for the rest of your life. And be prepared, because life-time changes to your health are not always easy. If it were easy, there wouldn't be so many unfit, unhealthy people wandering around hoping for a miracle pill to fix it all. So, picture yourself with the fit, lean, healthy body...the one you can truly admire (and that others will admire as well!). Then ask yourself 'how bad do you want it?' If the desire is there, you'll do the work. Maintain the vision of your goal – you as the ultimate Healthy Dude and stick with it!

But, before we get into what to eat and when, let's start at the end! And by that I mean your digestion and what happens to the food you eat. A better understanding of how your body actually uses food will make eating the right foods easier.

Digestion is more than just what happens in your stomach – there are actually ten organs that contribute to digesting and extracting nutrients from your food. The organs your food passes through: the mouth, pharynx, esophagus, stomach, small intestine, large intestine, anal canal/rectum. And, those that contribute to food breakdown: salivary glands, pancreas, and the liver and bile tract. My website at www.trishastewart.com gives a detailed description of each organ and its purpose, but for right now just understand that all of them work together to simplify (breakdown) the food you eat until it's in a form your body can absorb. That means it can pass through the walls of the intestines into the blood and lymph capillaries for circulation around the body. What's not usable is excreted through the bowels. While digestion simply happens without you thinking about it, it's a very complex system. If any part of the process is working inefficiently there will not be enough nutrients to support the body's cells.

So there are two ways to look at this, if the food you are eating is of poor quality and your digestive system is inefficient then this will lead to an inadequate supply of nutrients. On the other hand, if your digestive system has been compromised for some time, and you start to eat good quality food, your body will still not be able to absorb those nutrients for a while due to its lack of efficiency. So by eating junk, drinking too much alcohol and smoking you will find parts of this breaking down. Indigestion, constipation and diarrhea, bloating, wind and acid reflux are just a few signs that things are not working too well and it's time to examine your diet. What should you be eating? Great question! Let's take a look at the best things to eat for vitality and wellbeing.

Living Foods for Enzymes

Living foods like fruits and vegetables build and regenerate your body. When they're eaten fresh or raw (without cooking or preservatives) you get the most minerals, vitamins, carbohydrates, proteins (amino acids), fiber and enzymes they have to offer. I know there's a lot of focus on the amount of fats, carbohydrates and proteins you should eat, and I'm going to address that. But, first I want to talk about the key ingredient to good food – in any category – and that's enzymes. Enzymes are protein molecules with enormous health benefits.

The true life force of your body, enzymes are constantly breaking down and rejoining substances to rebuild and repair your body. Hidden within seeds and plants, they are the catalyst for the many thousands of chemical reactions that occur throughout the body; they are essential for the digestion and absorption of foods, as well as for the production of cellular energy. In other words, they are the element that enables the body to be nourished and live.

The absolute best way to ensure you get the enzymes, and therefore the nourishment, you need is eating raw, organic food which consists of vegetables, fruits, plants, seeds, nuts, sprouted grains, beans, and legumes. Heating food will destroy the enzymes and vitamins it holds. You see, once food reaches just over 100 degrees, the enzymes are killed and the food is, in essence, dead.

Now, I know many of you want to eat a hot, cooked meal and probably still will. But, it will be a great advantage to eat a raw salad before your main meal...even some grated carrots or other raw vegetables will help put some really great enzymes into your body, helping digestion and performing a host of other activities to help all those cells repair and renew. I would also suggest a raw snack in the middle of the morning or afternoon to up the amount of living food you're eating (a few carrot sticks, an apple or a handful of raw nuts). Now that you have the goal of eating more raw foods, let's take a closer look at what else you should be eating in more detail.

Proteins

Proteins play a vital role in the growth and repair of your body cells and tissues. They are also involved in the synthesis of enzymes, plasma (blood) proteins, antibodies (immune) and some hormones. And, they provide energy...although only after any available carbohydrates are burned. So, what are the best sources for protein? Believe it or not we do NOT need to eat meat, poultry, dairy, eggs or fish to get good quality protein. While you may have heard it's hard for vegetarians to get enough protein, I believe the best sources are in fact whole grains, nuts, seeds, beans, legumes, sea vegetables and some other vegetables. Plus, they're also classed as slow release or complex carbohydrates, so it is not hard to get all your protein, carbs and fiber in one meal!

I have already told you that I'm a vegetarian and promote that approach to diet. But, to you many life-time committed carnivores reading this, before you close this book and set it aside, please read a little further. The reason I do not promote the use of animal proteins is the information from several studies (many of which are referenced on my website www.trishastewart.com) that link eating meat to the following potential diseases and/irritating symptoms:

- Higher incidence of colorectal cancer
- Constipation leading to diverticulitis

- Higher incidences of colitis or other inflammatory digestive problem
- Headaches, bad breath
- Raised acidity leading to gall stones, liver damage, kidney stones and renal damage, bone loss/osteoporosis as the body excretes more calcium to maintain mineral balance
- Raised cholesterol
- Higher risk of heart disease
- Higher risk of diabetes or diabetic related symptoms
- Higher risk of obesity in adults and children
- Growth hormones and antibiotics used in mass producing cattle, sheep, pigs and poultry possibly causing infertility and who needs antibiotics!

For me it's clear, the benefits and increased vitality of a vegetarian lifestyle far exceed the risks of eating meat. Now I know you might not be able to cut out meat completely (or even want to...I get that). So, please, at least make the commitment to yourself to cut back...eat less fatty cuts and focus on organic meats...and increase your other sources of protein. Your body will thank you! And, just in case you are thinking you won't be able to build muscle without meat...check this out:

"I've never felt better. I'm healthier. I can train with more energy, and I'm not as much of a "hard guy" as I used to be. I've

become more concerned with my fellow man and the other inhabitants I share the planet with. ...I have now been vegetarian for almost 20 years. We have no fish, fowl, or red meat in our diet. Yet   I can still carry the same amount of muscle as I did in winning my four Mr. Universe titles. People can't believe it. They think that to have big muscles you have to eat meat - it's a persistent and recurring myth. But take it from me, there's nothing magic about eating meat that's going to make you a champion body builder. Anything you can find in a piece of meat, you can find in other foods as well."
Bill Pearl, Four-Time Mr. Universe

And get this! At the age of 41, Bill Pearl won the last Mr. Universe (1971)...weighing in at 242 lbs, with a height of 5'10" and 21" biceps!!

Another vegetarian bodybuilder is Steve Holt. At the age of 52 (he didn't even start training until his early 40's) he stood 5'8 ½", weight 165 pounds during competition and boasted 17" biceps and a 45" muscular chest. He placed in eight competitions over six years, usually taking 1st, 2nd or 3rd! So, if competitive bodybuilders can create great physiques eating a vegetarian diet, you can truly get into the best shape of your life doing the same thing!!

Carbohydrates

Carbohydrates are about energy...in fact, they are the easiest to digest, quickest source for giving you a shot of energy. That's why athletes often "carbo-load" before big games, races or events...for sustained energy. And, if you have carbohydrates providing the rapid energy and heat you need, your proteins can focus on repairing and rebuilding tissue (remember protein is burned AFTER all available carbs are used). That sounds simple enough, right? But, eating the wrong type of carbohydrates or any carbs eaten in excess can be stored as fat deposits under the skin (not great if you are trying to lose weight!). It can be a delicate balance to find the right amount of carbs for your body – enough to keep you energized and alert, but not too much to store as fat or make you lethargic.

How to make carbohydrates work for you!

Ideally, you want the slow release carbs from the starchy vegetables, grains and beans to help balance out the blood sugar levels. They release the sugars or glucose into the blood stream slowly...providing long-lasting, even energy. That's why oatmeal (a complex carb) in the morning is far more sustaining than crunchy cornflakes (made with simple carbs)!

Here's a quick list of sources for complex carbohydrates:

- Root vegetables like pumpkin, squash, carrot, beetroot/beets, sweet potato, white potato and corn.
- Low glycemic vegetables (that have little impact on blood sugar) including asparagus, aubergine/eggplant, broccoli, brussels sprouts, cabbage, cauliflower, celery, courgette/zucchini, cucumber, endive, fennel, garlic, kale, lettuce, mange tout/snow peas, mushrooms, onions, peas, peppers, radish, rocket, green beans, spinach, spring onions, tomatoes (technically a fruit) and watercress.

- Whole grains, rice, quinoa, buckwheat, millet, cornmeal, couscous, whole rye, whole wheat
- Legumes, lentils, peas, chick peas, split peas.
- Beans: soy, pinto, borlotti, butter, kidney, flageolet, haricot and black eyed peas
- Nuts and seeds, all kinds

This is just a partial list...check out www.trishastewart.com for a complete list.

Now, on the other hand, refined or simple carbs...such as all the white stuff (flour, rice, sugar, pasta, and bread), cookies, sticky buns, chocolate, sweets, puddings, ice cream and so on ... cause your blood sugar to rise rapidly. And, unless you are regularly exercising that means too much glucose in the blood stream so the body will dump it as fat deposits. Your blood sugar levels then crash and you will experience lethargy, poor concentration, palpitations and/or a feeling of anxiety and even sweating. And, here's the kicker...then you just crave more food, coffee and other stimulants...it's a vicious cycle! Believe it or not, years ago, even top athletes thought eating sweets (nothing but simple sugar) would give them a boost. Now, of course, we know that even though athletes don't dump excess sugars like sedentary folks, this was not and is not a good way to get energy. And, if simple carbs don't work well for active athletes, think about what they're doing to the masses of office bound workers who are eating them like they're going out of style. All those excess carbs means massive dumping of sugar or glucose into those fat deposits, or worse too much glucose in the blood system potentially causing diabetes and heart disease.

You probably know most of these things aren't good for you, but here's a list of those simple carbohydrates to avoid. I know, I know...they taste good!!! But, please think about what they're doing to your body...and how they are NOT delivering good nutrition.

- White bread, pasta (yes, it's just flour, water and sometimes a bit of egg), white rice, dinner rolls, buns, sweetened cereals and crackers
- Sweets, cookies, cakes, chocolates, soda pop, candy
- Frozen pizzas, microwave dinners, potato chips, roasted and salted nuts
- Sweetened fruit: canned fruits, jams, jellies and juices (yes, juice is from fruit, but all that concentrated fructose is still too much sugar)

The information on carbohydrates can be confusing, I know! You need to be wary of foods that provide nothing but "empty calories" as they lead to weight gain and feeling sluggish and tired. Get familiar with foods that have a minimal effect on your blood sugar level...

The following is the Glycemic Index table and description:

THE GLYCEMIC INDEX

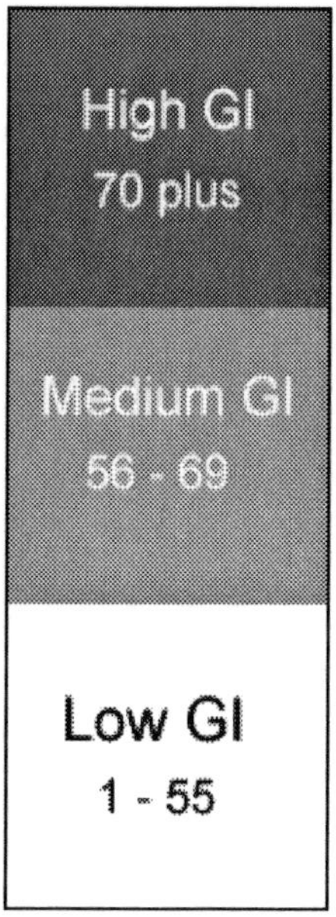

The GI or glycemic index is a system of measuring how different carbohydrate rich foods act on blood sugar levels. A rule of thumb is anything 55 or below because it will act slower therefore sustaining the blood sugar levels, ensuring a slow supply of energy.

The GL or glycemic load is another way of measuring. It lets us know the quality of the carbohydrate. For instance the carbohydrate of the watermelon has a high GI but there is not a lot of carbohydrate in the watermelon so the actual load or GL on the body is low. This means then that the watermelon will spike you up fairly quickly but it will not add too much carbohydrate into your diet.

We'll show more of this on the website as it's another way of working with your food. I'm not too keen on counting either calories or GI/GL but if you're not well, suffering from diabetes or have other reasons to know what your GI/GL is then it's a good way of monitoring your intake and knowing about both is very useful.

Glycemic Index (foods selected are based around what we are doing over the 30 days and of course beyond but a more comprehensive index will be available on the website.)

Food	grams	GI	GL
Whole oats	250	51	11
Pot Barley	150	25	11
Buckwheat	150	54	16
Polenta	150	69	9
Millet	150	71	25
Wholegrain Rice	150	55	18
Rice Noodles	180	61	23
Rice Cakes	25	78	17
Quinoa			
Butter beans	150	31	6
Black-eyed beans	150	42	13
Chick peas	150	28	8
Haricot beans	150	38	12
Red Kidney beans	150	28	7
Lentils	150	30	5
Pinto beans	150	39	10
Soya beans	150	18	1
Broad beans	80	79	9
Peas	80	48	3
Pumpkin	80	75	3
Sweetcorn	80	54	9
Beetroot	80	64	5
Carrots	80	47	3
Potatoes (white)	150	88	16 boiled
		85	26 baked
		75	22 fries
		91	18 mashed
Sweet Potato	150	44	11
Swede	150	72	7
Apple	120	38	6
Apricot	120	57	5

Food	grams	GI	GL
Banana	120	52	12
Grapes	120	49	9
Kiwi	120	53	6
Orange	120	42	5
Peach	120	42	5
Pears	120	38	4
Plum	120	39	5
Strawberries	120	40	1
Pineapple	120	66	6
Mango	120	51	8
Grapefruit	120	25	3
Cherries	120	22	3
Watermelon	120	72	4
Hummus	30	6	0
Cashew Nuts	50	22	3

FATS

You'd have to have been living under a rock to know that over the last 10 years people have been eating too much fat and oil. Not only does it naturally occur in the food you eat, but it's added to most of the packaged and prepared foods you buy. And, while some food companies and restaurants are taking steps to change that...it's really up to you to cut back. That should be easy, just avoid fatty foods wherever and whenever possible, right? Wrong. Eliminating too much fat is bad for you, because there are some oils and fats you need in your diet to keep healthy. So like good and bad proteins and carbohydrates...there are good and bad fats.

Not too long ago, there was an extreme low-fat diet craze that had people trying to cut out every type of fat in their diets. The problem? First, to make foods taste better the missing fat was usually replaced with sugar...and you've already read about what too much sugar does. So, low-fat diets actually make many people fat! Second, the lack of essential fats caused some serious health issues including symptoms of depression, ADHD, mental disturbances, schizophrenia, joint problems and more. So, what do you actually need?

Cholesterol.

Yes, believe it or not, you need cholesterol to help make bile to emulsify fat, synthesize sex hormones and protect the myelin sheath around the nerves. Sex hormones are **steroids** (fat soluble compounds) that control sexual maturity and reproduction. These **hormones** are produced mainly by the endocrine glands. The endocrine glands in females are ovaries and those in males are testes. While both males and females have all types of hormones present in their bodies, females produce the majority of two types of hormones, estrogens and progesterone, while males produce mainly androgens such as testosterone.

Most androgens produced by females are converted to estrogens and some androgens in males are also converted to estrogens. Sex hormones are synthesized from cholesterol (a fatty acid) and other compounds and secreted throughout a person's lifetime at different levels. Their production increases at puberty and normally decreases in old age. But, there's no need to take in any sources of cholesterol, your liver makes plenty to cover our required 2,000 mgs per day.

Unsaturated Fats.

Fat becomes an energy source when you have no carbohydrates stored, and it serves as padding to keep internal organs from bouncing around. Fats are also needed as protection around the nerves and to help keep cell membranes fluid so cells can change shape as needed, for instance, when red blood cells need to squeeze through capillaries. The problem is there are two types of fat...saturated and unsaturated. For a more detailed breakdown of fats - check out my website at: www.trishastewart.com, but here's a quick look. You need to avoid saturated fats that increase your blood cholesterol and body fat. Saturated fat includes butter, lard, bacon grease, margarine and solid (hydrogenated) vegetable shortening. On the other hand, unsaturated contain the essential fatty acids (or EFAs)...that's the type of fat your body needs. The best sources for EFAs are nut and seed oils and vegetable oils.

Here's another way to look at it. The fats from shellfish, dairy and red meat convert to prostaglandins which tend to increase inflammation in the body and encourage blood clotting. Those from vegetable, nut and seed oils tend to do the opposite. Some seed oils are more powerful in reducing inflammation and clotting than others. Flax (linseeds) contain the most 'omega-3' (and Omega 6) fatty acids which reduce blood clotting and reduce the risk for heart disease.

They are also particularly good at reducing joint inflammations like bursitis and the common form of arthritis called 'degenerative joint disease'. I recommend seed oil over fish oil primarily due to the inherent risk of toxins (like mercury) that can be present in certain fish (thanks to toxic pollution in our oceans). There are several particular seed oils I favor which contain a high amount of 'omega 3', omega-6 and omega-9' fatty acids good for reducing inflammation in the skin (eczema), and lungs (asthma)...Borage, blackcurrant, hemp, soy and flax seeds.

These oils have been particularly effective in reducing pain and inflammation from autoimmune diseases such as rheumatoid arthritis and lupus. However due to the highly unsaturated nature of these oils they can oxidize, causing free radical formation, which can cause inflammation and impaired immune function. That counteracts any benefits from taking the oil, so it's best to buy in small amounts.

Here's a guide to getting the right amount of fat every day: keep total fats down to 20% of calories. On a 1500 calorie diet, that means 300 calories from fat per day, preferably a seed oil or seeds and nuts. Consume omega-3, 6 and 9 fats through flax and other seeds and nuts. If you have a specific health problem, try using an essential fatty acid supplement such as those mentioned above, plus an antioxidant nutrient.

What about vitamins and minerals?

If you're eating a proper diet, I feel taking additional supplements is usually unnecessary. However, if you're under a tremendous amount of stress (which will burn out vitamins and minerals), on any medication, sick, find eating difficult, or burning up everything you eat (athletes) additional supplements may be needed. And, for people on the go who need an occasional boost to the body, I would suggest a twice yearly supplementation. For more information on my Six-Monthly Body Boost and why I recommend "superfoods" visit my website at www.trishastewart.com.

The 30-Day Detox

Okay, so I've given you information on food groups and sources, and even a few key foods and things to avoid. So, by now you're probably thinking...okay, Trisha what exactly should I be eating...I need more specifics. Well, let's get to it. The best way for you to get on track with eating right is to use my 30-Day Detox plan. It's an effective way to rid your body of any toxins and junk from bad eating habits. Then, you can build from these basic menus to create your own customized eating plan. And, for a quick easy reference, I've included a basic shopping list at the end of this chapter. But, before you stock your cupboards from the shopping list, start with the 30-Day Detox and plan your shopping around what you actually need.

The 30-Day Plan to Reach Eden

The 30-Day Plan is broken down into 5 sections. This plan is very doable...NO starvation...no constant hunger...no feeling faint. Each section carefully prepares you for the next phase and ultimately for getting your health and vitality back for keeps. The 30-day Plan breaks down as follows:

- o   7 days – gentle detox
- o   5 days – light food
- o   2 days- juicing
- o   7 days – light food
- o   9 days – light food with introduction of certain other foods

A few notes to keep in mind during the next 30-days

- •   I have allowed light frying of foods, but remember to be careful how you fry or sauté. Use stocks and other liquids or the smallest amounts of approved oils.
- •   Eat organic wherever possible
- •   The foods are vegetarian/vegan because they will be less taxing on the body systems and organs and will help to raise the Ph or alkalinity.

- I have tried to create a program with a lot of variety and different foods for you to try, but don't feel you have to eat things you don't enjoy. You can focus on wholesome vegetable and bean soup, a juice, oats or muesli...but vary the ingredients and at least try a few new things.

- Try and be a bit more adventurous with the evening meal particularly at the weekend when you have time, experiment with different herbs, spices, vegetables etc and be creative. Feed more than your body...feed your soul.

- If you wish to swap your lunch for your evening meal this is okay and actually better for you.

- Check your bowels. They should be moving at least once a day...preferably more. If things are not 'moving', increase your fluids or visit my website (www.TrishaStewart.com) for personalized help. And, for a quick reference...revisit Chapter Three.

- Your urine will probably be quite colored and smelly for a day or so, but this will clear.

- You may go through what we term a "healing crisis" whereby you may get headaches, nausea and maybe a little feverish, and get facial or body spots. This will last for a maximum of 72 hours. It's just your body adjusting to the changes and trying to eliminate toxins out of every orifice. If this does happen increase your fluid intake and rest when possible. The best time to start your 30-day plan is over a weekend if you are working, by Monday you will be raring to go.

- Remember, this is not like any of the quick fix detox plans. This is a way of eating that you can always come back to and should in the long term. I do not propose any quick fix...that is merely sticking a small band aid over a major wound. I am talking life long health, so these changes to your eating can be implemented every day or your life. This is a healthy way to eat long term. But I do know the other foods will creep in so you can always come back to Step 8 or sooner if you begin to loose the vitality that you will gain over the next 30 days and beyond.

- At this stage we will use products that will enhance the cleansing and healing process rather than add vitamins and minerals. The main reason is that your gut will probably be compromised at this stage and not absorbing as well as it will in a short time. And, as long as you're eating a good, balanced organic diet...I don't believe in long term use of supplements anyway. However, you may find benefits with these supplements:

  1. Acidophilus culture. Lactobacillus acidophilus in capsule or powdered form will add good bacteria to the intestines and bowel and help in controlling the bad bacteria.

  2. Milk Thistle, great for supporting the liver

3. Omega 3,6,9 from seed oil for helping to reduce inflammation and calms the nervous system

4. MSM a great sulfur rich cleanser for the whole system

5. Check out the "superfoods" on my website

- Cut the following from your diet eating only the foods I have suggested on the 30 day plan:
    1. Yeast in bread, rolls, pizza, gravy powders, marmite, etc.
    2. Wheat, cereals and ready-made products
    3. Cut out all sugar, that which you add and that which is already added. i.e. biscuits, cakes, chocolate, sweets, ice creams, puddings, chewing gum, sweeteners and anything that says it is sugar free but has a sweetener in it.
    4. Fruit consumption is to be pears and apples only in the initial phase (no dried fruits in muesli or eaten on their own)
    5. No added salt or very minimal pure sea salt
    6. No takeaways, ready meals, fast foods, etc.
    7. All meat, game and poultry, fish, eggs
    8. Coffee, tea, hot chocolate, etc.
    9. All dairy foods
    10. Refined grains i.e. those not with the hull, bran and germ intact

11. All alcohol

12. Smoking (if possible PLEASE!)

13. Over the counter medicines

14. And, finally check with your doctor to make sure you are not being over-prescribed medication.

- Eat plenty of the following foods freely

1. All vegetables/salads/herbs raw or cooked

Fresh vegetable juices anytime

Keep a pan of soup ready for quick snacks and meals

Have some crudités ready for nibbling or dipping into hummus, guacamole and other dips (I've included a few dip recipes)

2. Nuts and seeds

3. Pears, avocado, apples. Other fruits in season but limited for the first seven days

4. Whole grains such as wholegrain rice, quinoa, millet, buckwheat, oats, etc.

5. Sprouted beans, seeds etc.

6. Breakfast oats, millet, quinoa

7. Tofu or other soy bean products (not ready made sausages/burgers etc as they will contain salt, flavorings and preservatives

8. Soy yogurt and milk

9. Nut milks or rice milk
10. Nut butters (check out my recipes for healthy ones).

- Fluids to include
  1. Filtered spring or distilled water hot or cold
  2. Fruit or herbal teas
  3. Chinese Green teas

NOTE: Any of the menu items below that have an asterisk (*) means I have included the recipe in the following section.

Seven days – Gentle Detox

- Start each day with a pint(2½ cups) of hot water with lemons and limes infused or two tablespoons apple cider vinegar
- Mid-morning and mid-afternoon have crudités with a dip (mid-morning) and a handful of nuts and seeds (mid-afternoon) or in reverse according to what you fancy. Or, have a bowl of light vegetable soup
- Choose from the recipes but try and balance out your foods in the following ways

Monday

Breakfast: Healthy Dude Oatmeal* topped with fresh or stewed pears or apples. You may add vanilla pods, cinnamon or nutmeg to taste or the homemade muesli.

Lunch: Healthy Dude Veggie Salad: Mixed leaf salad with sprouts, nuts and seeds, avocado, grated beetroot/beets, celery, courgette, grated carrot and cherry tomatoes. Make a dressing from olive oil, lemon/lime juice, crushed garlic plus any herbs you may flavor, shake it all up in a jar.

Dinner: Enjoy lots of different vegetables and beans to serve with whole grain rice or quinoa and add into a curry, chili (use fresh chili if possible far nicer flavor than powder) or a casserole. Choose from the recipes

Tuesday

Breakfast: Stewed pears/apples and natural soy yogurt flavored with nutmeg, vanilla, topped with nuts and seeds or homemade muesli

Lunch: *Simple homemade carrot and coriander soup with a mixed leaf salad & sprouts

Dinner: *Tofu and bean burgers with mixed vegetables selection and homemade sweet potato wedges and a dip of your choice from included recipes

Wednesday

Breakfast: Breakfast as usual or *buckwheat pancakes with stewed fruit folded inside plus a juice from the recipes

Lunch: Quinoa and veggie salad with a *spicy dressing

Dinner: *Provencal stew, rice pasta or polenta with a green salad to include baby leaf spinach, parsley, lambs lettuce, beet greens or whatever you fancy

Thursday

Breakfast: *Lentil patties with lightly sautéed tomatoes plus a juice from any of the recipes

Lunch: Homemade soup with a mixed salad of sprouts and leaves

Dinner: *Poached Tofu in a Thai sauce, garlic potatoes, steamed spinach or kale, carrots and fresh peas

Friday

Breakfast: Oat or millet porridge or homemade muesli with apples and pears

Lunch: *Wholegrain rice and root vegetable with a dressing (cold or hot)

Dinner: *Bean casserole topped with potatoes; serve with green vegetables in season

Saturday

Breakfast: Apples and pears with natural soy yogurt and nutmeg

Lunch: Baked sweet potato with ratatouille

Dinner: *Vegetable paella (can be used as it is or to stuff peppers, aubergines/eggplant or any other vegetable you can stuff)

Sunday

Breakfast: Sauté potatoes, mushrooms, tomatoes and onions

Lunch: Large green salad with a selection of other vegetables home made coleslaw

Dinner: *Nut roast with an onion gravy, green vegetables, roasted roots

I realize this may not sound like much of a detox, but believe me you will have missed your bread, sugar and...for meat eaters...your flesh foods. But, you will feel a whole lot better, probably lost a few pounds and will have renewed energy. Keep going. Did I hear anyone say they had no indigestion this week and bowel movements were good? Check these daily! If not, your digestion is more compromised than you thought. Keep going and check the website for more information and support www.TrishaStewart.com).

Five Days - Light Food

Ok so you have now completed seven really important days, seven days that will enhance the rest of your life. The next five days will remain very similar but with the inclusion of other fruits which will be juiced or eaten whole plus a two day only, weekend of juicing. Try to eat with the seasons so whatever fruit is available but limit grapes and banana and if using melon do not have it with other fruits, eat it alone. Keep these pointers in mind:

- Keep up with the fluids as before
- If you can grow some sprouts this week, even if it is only alfalfa that would be great for your juices and of course added to any other foods
- Don't forget to drink a pint (2 ½ cups) of hot water with lemon and limes or apple cider vinegar as soon as you rise from your bed and to drink at least two liters more during the day

Monday

Breakfast: Make a breakfast juice of apples, carrot, celery, parsley, spinach, pineapple and a little natural soy yogurt if you like the texture smooth and creamy

Lunch: Seasonal vegetable soup with beans and a leafy salad

Dinner: *Red peppers stuffed with spicy vegetables served with greens

Tuesday

Breakfast: Breakfast juice as before with maybe some variation according to what you enjoy and what is in season

Lunch: Seasonal vegetable soup with beans and a leafy salad

Dinner: Tofu and vegetable Thai curry with wholegrain rice and raita

Wednesday

Breakfast: Oats with apples and pears or a juice or both if you feel hungry

Lunch: *Tabouleh with a green salad

Dinner: *Parsnip and carrot risotto with wilted spinach

Thursday

Breakfast: Juice plus oat or millet porridge or homemade muesli

Lunch: Beetroot/beets cooked and sliced, red onion sliced thinly, crumbled walnuts sat on top of a large leafy salad, all the herb leaves as well as usual lettuce leaves and herbs plus a dressing

Dinner: *Lentil dhal and roasted garlic with spinach or other greens

Friday

Breakfast: Juice as before

Lunch: Large bowl of season soup with a side salad

Dinner: Parsnip, chickpeas with onions, *chili and ginger sauce, quinoa, and raita

Two Days - Juicing

By now your body should be working a lot more efficiently, your kidneys, bladder, bowels and liver should be really flushing, emptying and processing, what a great job you have done! But now brace yourselves for juicing. If you can't manage to just juice please add in some soups instead of or as well as. I am not letting you off the hook here, but if you REALLY cannot face it please go to two of the days the previous week and repeat the menu but I have to tell you if you are on a weight loss track this will certainly help to drop a few more pounds.

You will need to relax and have a chill out weekend. Ensure you have scheduled this in, you have had plenty of time to do so, no excuses, and this is your life! It's a great time to do a salt scrub and an Epsom salt bath (not if you have high blood pressure though please), or a gentle bath in some essential oils and some skin brushing.

Okay, here's the basic juice program. You will have five juices daily, plus masses of filtered water and soups...but only vegetable soups. No grains or beans to be added to the soup. Note that some of the juice recipes are for one person, please increase accordingly for more people.

Day One:

On rising have a pint of hot water with lemon/lime slices or apple cider vinegar. Then make the following juices (with your juicer...remember not a blender or smoothie maker).

8am juice	Two apples, stick of celery, handful of spinach or kale, ¼ pineapple, ½ ripe avocado
11am juice	Two apples, Medium carrot, handful mixed leaves (kale, spinach, parsley) ½ medium sized beetroot/beets, ¼ lemon, ginger to taste, alfalfa sprouts
2pm juice	Similar to the 11am juice but add in anything that you feel like to go with it, maybe avocado or cucumber or broccoli or some other herbs
5pm juice	Two apples, one pear, ½ pineapple, handful of greens, stick of celery, ¼ avocado, chunk courgette/zucchini
8pm	Make this a nice smoothie for relaxing at the end of the day. Half avocado, some fruits of your choice including half of a banana

Before bed if you feel like it, stew some apples and add cinnamon.

Day Two:

Repeat the same idea on Sunday but have a supper of chunky vegetable soup with beans. You should be raring to go on Monday so up you get, a pint (2 ½ cups) of hot water with lemons/limes or apple cider vinegar, have your mid morning and mid afternoon snacks as usual.

7 Days - Light Food

For the next week, you will have a mixture of the previous two weeks. Keep in mind all of the previous notes about water intake and starting each day with a pint of hot water with the usual additions. You can change up the menu a bit to suit your tastes.

Monday

Breakfast: Fruit and natural soy yogurt with nuts and seeds or a juice of your choice or both

Lunch: Big chunky soup with side salad

Dinner: *Simple root veggie hotpot with green vegetables and homemade potato wedges, with a dip of your choice from the provided recipes

Tuesday

Breakfast: Juice for breakfast

Lunch: Spicy lentil and bean salad with a leafy salad

Dinner: Tofu, vegetable and cashew nut sir fry with a *ginger and chili sauce, serve with wholegrain rice or quinoa

Wednesday

Breakfast: Oat or millet porridge or homemade muesli with
              fresh fruit and/or a juice

Lunch: Large salad with lots of different
              vegetables/leaves, tomatoes, basil or other herb
              dressing, avocado, nuts and seeds and sprouts and
              olives

Dinner: *No meat shepherds pie with carrots and greens

Thursday

Breakfast: Juice and *Tofu scramble

Lunch: Chunky soup and salad

Dinner: Vegetable and chickpea curry with wholegrain rice
              or quinoa and raita

Friday

Breakfast: Oat or millet porridge or homemade muesli with
              fruit and/or juice

Lunch: Sliced avocado, thinly sliced onions, sliced
              tomatoes, sliced cucumber, topped with hummus
              and olives

Dinner: Roasted root salad with whole garlic, marinated
              tofu and homemade coleslaw

Saturday

Breakfast: Potato cakes, mushrooms, tomatoes, onions

Lunch: Jacket potato with a spice bean filling or
              ratatouille

Dinner: *Pasta with a red pepper sauce and a huge salad

Sunday
Breakfast: Juice, muesli

Lunch: *Stuffed peppers and a leafy salad

Dinner: Lentil Dhal with fried vegetable rice and wilted
spinach

Hopefully this week has worked wonders for your digestive
system and your energy will have increased yet again.

9 Days - Light food & Extras

The following and last days of your 30-day plan will include a
couple of little extras... not much though, so don't get too
excited. Instead, be excited about how you are feeling...your
renewed energy, clear skin and eyes. I bet your nails have
grown also. Check in with yourself to see how you really feel
and what has changed, note the changes in your journal, and
give yourself a pat on the back for doing so well.

The following seven days will include all of the foods you have
eaten before but you may have some oat cakes, rice cakes,
corn crackers to have with your mid-morning snack. I will do a
"pick and mix" of the recipes so that you eat a variety of
beans, grains, legumes, tofu, etc. Saturday and Sunday will
include foods that you may have periodically during the weeks

ahead such as tortilla wraps or soda bread, sourdough, flatbreads etc. But please be aware they may upset your tummy so don't eat too much.

Breakfast each day

> Healthy Dude Oatmeal* with fruit, Healthy Dude Muesli*, plus juice from the recipes or from the Healthy Bunch Cookbook

Snacks each day

You can now include a couple of oat cakes with some hummus or guacamole or nuts/seeds or a bowl of light vegetable soup.

Monday

Lunch: Large salad with grated roots vegetables, avocado, walnuts, cherry tomatoes and a dressing

Dinner: *Teriyaki style tofu with Asian noodles

Tuesday

Lunch: Seasonal soup with corn crackers

Dinner: Chickpea curry served with wholegrain rice

Wednesday

Lunch: Tabbouleh served on a bed of leaves

Dinner: Tofu Thai style, plus a wholegrain and greens of your choice

Thursday

Lunch: Jacket Potato stuffed with chili, ratatouille or other favorite

Dinner: Provencal stew with rice pasta or polenta and greens

Friday

Lunch: Seasonal soup and oatcakes

Dinner: Tofu Burgers, potato wedges, salad, plus a dip of your choice from the provided recipes

Saturday

Lunch: Avocado salad

Dinner: Carrot and parsnip risotto with spinach or other greens

Sunday

Lunch: Potato rosti with dips and a salad

Dinner: Nut roast with a red onion sauce, green vegetables and roast potatoes

From here on...

- Once every other day you can include any yeast free bread, preferably rye flour or sourdough, tortilla wraps, oat cakes, rice cakes (all sugar, yeast and preservative free so probably best to make them or purchase them from a very good supplier)

- Vary the vegetables raw and cooked, the grains and pulses see shopping list or the good bad and ugly if you want to make sure you are doing it right
- Carnivores please try to keep to a minimum of meat, poultry, game and fish, please choose organic where possible but hopefully you will have enjoyed the vegetarian foods so much your tastes will have changed forever.

At the end of these 30 days you're going to feel better than ever...more energy, more stamina, probably even lost some weight, and now you have an idea of how to eat your way to optimum health – one day at a time. But, there are a few more things to be wary of – and downright avoid. Along with sugars (real and artificial), which I've touched on when talking about carbohydrates, you need to know more about alcohol and cheese...those fermented popular goodies and the "the good, the bad and the ugly" foods. So, if you want to know what really goes on when you eat them, sign up on my website at www.trishastewart.com.

Recipes for the 30-day Plan

Look out for my book, The Healthy Bunch Cookbook, for a much expanded range of healthy vegetarian recipes.

Healthy Dude Porridge

This can be a small cupful of oats to 2 cups of water or a mix of water and soy or rice milk. Put in a small pan, just bring to simmer for a few minutes, add more fluid if necessary. It will depend on the size of the oats as to how much fluid.

You can make millet or quinoa porridge in exactly the same way but may need to vary the fluid

Or make a mix of oats, millet and quinoa.

You can add to this the following:

1. Pure vanilla essence or a vanilla pod
2. Nutmeg
3. Cinnamon
4. Nuts and Seeds, ground or whole
5. Fresh stewed fruit
6. A little soy yogurt

Oatcakes

350g (about 1½ cups)of fine oatmeal or coarse if you like a rustic oatcake

1 tsp of good quality sea salt

150ml (2/3 cup) boiling water

50ml (1¾ oz) of olive oil, walnut or other oil (may need to check consistency and add more) you can also use Tahini, Nut butter or any Vegan Butter that will melt.

Pinch of bicarbonate of soda

Mix everything together and turn out onto a board, knead and roll out into two big rounds. Make some cuts across to form triangles and bake on a tray which has been oiled. Bake in a cool oven of around 300 F/150C/gas mark 2 for about one hour, do not overcook or they will be too hard.

Healthy Dude Muesli

½ cup each of oats, rice flakes and millet. Add chopped nuts, sunflower seeds, sesame seeds, pumpkin seeds and flax seeds. Soak in soy or rice milk for half an hour or less - if you like the mixture a little dry then top with soy (natural) yogurt and fresh fruit.

Savory millet, lentil and brazil nut loaf

125g (1/2 cup) millet, 125g (2/3 cup) green lentils, sprouted, 1 cup vegetable stock or mineral water, 1 tablespoon tapioca flour, 125g (1/2 cup) roughly chopped brazil nuts, 2 sticks celery, 1 tablespoon fresh sage.

Preheat oven to 150 C (310 F) or gas 3, cook millet and lentils in the stock or mineral water and mix with rest of ingredients, oil loaf tin or deep pie dish and press mixture well in, bake for 45 minutes or until top of loaf is brown and firm to touch.

Simple carrot and coriander soup (use other vegetables and herbs in to create your own Homemade Soup)

Use 1 lb of carrots to 1½ pints (3 ¾ cups) of yeast free vegetable stock (cube will do but use low salt one).

Put a small amount of olive oil into base of large pan, put in one chopped onion, clove of garlic and sweat (on low with lid on) for a few minutes. Add chopped carrots plus a large chopped sweet potato plus one leek (optional). Pour on stock, bring to boil then turn down and simmer until cooked. Add fresh bunch of coriander. When cooled I like to blend three parts and leave some chunky bits in, but this is your choice, blend all or none if preferred.

Quick Tofu and Bean Burgers

Makes 6-8

1 medium onion, peeled and chopped

1 large peeled garlic clove or to taste

1 medium carrot, peeled and coarsely grated (about 60g prepared weight)

420g (15 oz) can 'no-salt no-sugar' red kidney beans, drained and rinsed in a colander under cold running water or a mix of other beans

220g pack smoked or natural tofu, drained

75g (1/3 cup) sunflower seeds

1 small bunch parsley (about 20g)

2 tsp organic wheat and yeast free vegetable bouillon powder

Preheat the oven to 220C/Gas Mark 7. Line a large baking tray with baking parchment Place all the ingredients in a food processor and blend roughly do not puree. If you don't have a food processor, crumble or mash the tofu and beans and add to the other ingredients.

Grab a handful of mixture and form into a ball and place on the baking tray. Press with fingertips to make a burger shape, how many you will get depends on the size burger you would like. Bake for 25 minutes, do not overcook, these are great hot or cold or served with a creamy sauce.

Buckwheat Pancakes

This is a basic recipe; you may like to play around with different ingredients to make this work for you. They will not be as light as the usual pancakes as you are using different flour.

1 heaped cup buckwheat flour

2 + teaspoons baking powder

Pinch of pure sea salt

1 cup soy milk, rice milk or almond milk

1 teaspoon pure vanilla essence

2 Tablespoons ground almonds or finely chopped walnuts

For variety you can add nut butters such as almond or seeds butter such as Tahini (sesame) when blending the wet ingredients.

Beat it all together and ladle into a frying pan which has hot olive or sunflower oil in it.

Provencal Stew

1 large onion, chopped

Garlic and olive oil, to taste

1 large aubergine/eggplant, cut into cubes (salted, drained, and blotted dry if desired)

2 red peppers, sliced

3 large tomatoes, seeded and chopped

2 courgette/zucchini, chopped

Salt and pepper to taste

Herbs de Provence dried which should be a mix of Rosemary, Basil, Marjoram, Savory, and Thyme. I also like to put in fresh Basil it has such a wonderful smell and taste, add towards the end.

- Sauté onion and garlic in olive oil
- Add the aubergine/eggplant and fry a few minutes.
- Add the peppers, tomatoes and zucchini.
- Add herbs to taste.
- Let cook over medium-low heat for 30 minutes, stirring occasionally.

Serve hot as a main dish, or cold as a side dish.

This is a very handy recipe as you can stuff it into jacket (sweet or white) potato, or stuff any vegetable that is "stuffable."

Lentil Rissoles

Cup dry lentils, (red/green/brown) cooked in 2 cups water

1 cup carrots, shredded or finely diced

1 medium onion, finely chopped

1 cup red or green pepper finely diced

1 courgette/zucchini finely diced

2 cups medium/fine oats

1/4 cup extra virgin olive oil

3/4 cup tomato paste

1 tablespoon Italian seasoning

- Bring water to boil and put lentils in, bring back to simmer for about 15 minutes or until just soft.
- Sauté the onions in a frying/sauté pan until they look translucent, do not brown
- Add peppers and courgette/zucchini cook until just softening
- Put the ingredients in a bowl and add the lentils and bind together
- Shape them into rolls, rounds, squares or whatever suits you.

You can add spices to these for a change and try different vegetables such as celery or spinach, sweet potato mashed with the lentil mixture, they are great hot or cold.

Poached Tofu and Thai Sauce

2 Sweet red chilies seeded and chopped

1 lemon grass stalk chopped

1inch piece of ginger root, peeled and chopped finely

2 Kaffir Lime Leaves

1 bunch fresh coriander (cilantro)

1 tsp ground coriander

(If the above ingredients are not available use dried, it will
not be as nice and you will have to blend to taste)

1 pack of Tofu, (plain, smoked or herb) cubed or sliced

- Put all the above ingredients (except the Tofu) into
  a food processor or use a pestle and mortar and
  blend
- Add 400ml (1 2/3 cups) of coconut milk to the
  above and mix together
- Place in a frying or sauté pan and add the Tofu and
  simmer so that the ingredients can come together
  in flavor, about 20 minutes or more if preferred.

Bean Casserole

2 large onions sliced

Little olive oil

2 cloves garlic diced (or to taste)

1" piece of ginger sliced or diced

4 Tomatoes sliced

½ courgette/zucchini sliced

4 Tbsp Tahini

500ml (2 cups) vegetable stock from yeast free bouillon or
homemade stock

Mixed beans such as Haricot, Kidney, Flageolet, Butter (cooked) if using tinned ensure sugar and salt free and rinse thoroughly

2 tsp mixed dried herbs such as Italian or Provence

1 Large Sweet Potato sliced

Fresh herbs to dress

- In a large sauté pan, put a little olive oil and sauté the sliced onions till transparent
- Add the garlic and ginger, sauté for a minute or two
- Add the tomatoes and courgette/zucchini
- Add the beans
- Mix the Tahini, herbs and vegetable stock and add to the mixture, do not make it too wet at this stage
- Put into a casserole dish
- Place the sweet potato on top
- Bake in the oven on 170c 325f gas 3 for about an hour

You can leave it all in the sauté pan, put the potato on top and simmer with a lid on, baked in the oven is nicer though

You may need to add a little stock if the casserole gets to look dry

Vegetable paella (fast version)

Portion of cooked wholegrain rice

1 large sliced onion

1 clove garlic sliced or diced

1 stick celery sliced

1 carrot cut into sticks

1 red or green pepper cut into slices

1 courgette/zucchini cut into sticks

Handful of mange tout/snowpeas left whole or sliced

Yeast free vegetable stock

- In a large flat frying pan sauté some garlic, onions and celery in olive oil for 5 minutes
- Add sticks of carrot, peppers, courgette/zucchini, mange tout or any vegetables you like.
- Add the rice
- Add the stock to taste, not too wet
- Add pine nuts, broken cashew nuts, olives and serve with green salad.

The above paella ingredients are ideal to stuff peppers, aubergine/eggplant and any other 'stuffable' vegetables.

If you want to make the longer version, add uncooked risotto rice, about 1 cup to the onions, garlic and celery mix, then add the vegetables and ladle in the stock so that the rice can cook, this is a little time consuming but very nice although I do find risotto rice very starchy compared to wholegrain, so not ideal.

Nut Roast

1tbs extra-virgin olive oil

3 cups of mixed nuts, ground or finely chopped

12 oz tomatoes, blanched, peeled & chopped or tinned

1 large onion

1 clove garlic diced

1/4lb fresh mushrooms, chopped

1/2 tsp dried basil and dried oregano or other mixed herbs to taste

1 - 1/2 cups of cooked millet or quinoa

Directions

- Preheat oven to 425 F (220) gas 7
- Lightly oil a loaf tin
- Sauté the onion and garlic in a little olive oil until the onion is transparent
- Place these in a mixing bowl and add the rest of the ingredients
- Turn the mixture into the prepared loaf tin, smoothing the surface with the back of a spoon. Place the tin in oven and bake for 30-40 minutes

Serve with onion gravy made from sliced onions sautéed in olive oil, 1 1/2 cups of vegetable stock, 1 tbsp tomato paste, 1 tsp mustard, bring to a simmer until cooked.

Tabbouleh

1 cup of bulgur wheat

1 ½ cups of boiling water

3 tbsp lemon juice

1 clove garlic grated or crushed in a pestle and mortar

Bunch of fresh mint chopped or ½ tsp dried

¾ tbsp olive oil

4 to 6 spring onions chopped (use the green if nice)

3 tomatoes diced

1 small cucumber diced

½ cup of olives if liked

Bunch parsley some chopped some left for garnish

- Combine the bulgur wheat and water, stir and let sit for 30 minutes to re-hydrate
- Stir after the 30 minutes to check there is no moisture, if there is drain off
- Add lemon juice, garlic and oil
- Add the remaining ingredients and stir

This is nice if left to sit for a while so that the flavors can combine.

Parsnip and Carrot Risotto

1 ½ cups of dry rice (check with the paella recipe for the fast or slow version)

1 large sliced onion

1 clove garlic diced

2 or 3 carrots cut into sticks

1 or 2 parsnips cut into sticks

1 liter or more of yeast free vegetable stock

Bunch Fresh coriander chopped (or other fresh herbs)

Olive oil

- Sauté the onion in a little olive oil with the garlic
- Add the uncooked rice (if doing the slow version)
- Add the parsnip and carrots
- Ladle in the stock to allow the rice and vegetables to cook in a little of the liquid, adding more as ingredients begin to dry
- Just towards the end add the fresh coriander or other herbs

If doing the fast version and using cooked rice, add this just before the vegetables are cooked and then add the stock to taste do not make too wet. This does not hurt to simmer slowly until you are ready to eat.

Red Lentil Dhal

Olive oil

1 tsp garlic, crushed

1 tsp each fresh chili and ginger, finely chopped and mixed

2 tsp powdered turmeric

1 tsp garam masala

1 tsp ground coriander

2 tbsp fresh coriander, finely chopped

1 cinnamon stick

1 tsp mustard

1 large whole tomato, diced finely

1 medium onion, diced finely

2 sticks celery, diced finely

800ml/27 oz water

225g (1 cup) red lentils, washed well

- Heat the oil in a saucepan with a thick base
- Add garlic, chili, ginger and spices (except fresh coriander) and herbs, mustard, tomato, onion and celery.
- Fry for about 10 minutes until well blended.e
- Add the water and bring to the boil
- Stir the lentils in and cook on a low heat for about half an hour, until the lentils are soft, stirring occasionally.

You may need to add a little stock or water if the dhal becomes dry. If you have time place a couple of bulbs of garlic in the oven and roast for half an hour, take out and press the juicy roasted garlic and add to the dhal, some chopped almonds on top are nice and also the fresh coriander.

This is a good side dish for a vegetable curry, good on its own with some homemade spicy onion koftas.

Stir Fried Greens, Ginger and Oyster Sauce

1lb Chinese greens, pak choy/bok choy, and baby spinach

1 tablespoon walnut oil

1 tablespoon sesame oil

1" sliced fresh ginger

1 fresh red chili sliced

4 spring onions

2 tablespoons oyster sauce (no added sugar)

¼ yeast free stock cube make up a with a little water

Juice of ½ lemon and some black pepper

- Blanche pak choy/bok choy for 1 minute in boiling water and drain.
- In large wok fry ginger and onions in oils, add rest of ingredients, add oyster sauce, stock cube and lemon juice.
- If you want more sauce add water and thicken with potato starch.
- Serve with rice noodles or rice or quinoa.

Raita relish, dip or condiment

200 ml (8 oz) soy yogurt

1/8 tsp cumin powder

Pinch paprika

½ cup cucumber finely diced

1 tsp. finely crushed coriander leaves

- Whisk the yogurt
- Add the other ingredients
- Garnish with fresh coriander

To ring the changes try using finely diced tomato, onion, cooked potato, blanched shredded spinach or other vegetable you like.

Simple Root Vegetable Hotpot

- Sauté/sweat a chopped onion and garlic in a pan
- Add a variety of chopped vegetables (about 1 1/2 lb), some tinned tomatoes, herbs and a half pint of water with some yeast free stock and a little tomato puree. Simmer gently or put in the oven.

Make sure that the hot pot does not dry; you may need a little more water depending on vegetables used. Add some cooked lentils or other pulses/beans to make a more substantial meal.

Tofu, vegetable and cashew nut stir fry (serve with rice or other grain)

1 pack Tofu, cubed

1 large onion sliced

1 garlic clove diced

1 inch piece of ginger root diced or grated

2 fresh sweet chilies, de-seeded and chopped finely

A mix of thinly sliced vegetables such as carrot, green or red peppers, celery, zucchini/courgette, mange tout/snowpeas or fresh peas (any you fancy)

Cashew Nuts

- Heat a small amount of olive oil in a wok or large frying pan
- Add tofu and lightly fry till golden brown, then remove.

- Add the onion and garlic, chili and ginger, sauté for a few minutes
- Put in a mixture of thinly sliced carrots, green pepper, ginger, celery etc and sauté for 1 min to mix flavors
- Add some cashews
- Add a little yeast free stock; put in the tofu and sauté all vegetables until they are as soft as you would like them.

No meat Shepherd's Pie

110g (4oz) brown lentils

900g (2lbs) potatoes, roughly chopped

3 tbsp olive oil

3-5 tbsp soy milk

8oz onions or leeks sliced

4oz carrots, small slices

4oz parsnips, small slices

8oz mushrooms, roughly chopped

3-4 sticks celery, sliced

2 tbsp tomato puree

225g (8oz) chopped tomatoes, fresh or tinned

1tbsp soy sauce

1/8tsp rosemary

1tsp dried oregano

- Cook the lentils in stock or water until they are tender (about 1 hour).

- Cook the potatoes in boiling salted water. When tender, drain and mash with the milk to obtain creamy (not sloppy) mashed potatoes. Season to taste.
- Meanwhile sauté the onions, celery, carrots and parsnips with a small amount of olive oil, until almost tender. If they are slow in cooking, add a bit of water, cover and cook until the carrots are tender.
- Add the mushrooms and continue to cook until they are softening, then add the lentils, tomatoes, tomato puree, oregano and rosemary and cook for a few more minutes. Season to taste with soy sauce and salt and pepper.

  Spread out in an ovenproof dish. Cover with mashed potatoes about 2cm thick. Bake at 200C (375F, gas 5) for 30-40 minutes

Tofu Scramble

This is one of those simple recipes to make with a variation to suit so try your own.

The basis is 1 pack Tofu

1 small onion finely diced

A little diced garlic

Red pepper, courgette/ zucchini, whatever you have diced

A little turmeric or cumin or other spices or herbs that you like

A little olive oil to fry in

- Drain, cube and crumble the Tofu

- Sauté off the onion, garlic, spices or herbs (if fresh leave till last)
- Add your choice of vegetables cook till you like the consistency

Quick Bean Salad - add some mixed salad leaves and rice or other grain

Mix a variety of dried, cooked beans such as kidney, borlotti, black eye, flageolet with some lightly steamed French, broad or runner beans and mixed fresh herbs, olive oil and lemon/lime juice. You can buy tinned beans for emergencies but ensure sugar and salt free.

Adding curry spices to this makes a change.

Quick Rice and lentil salad - add some mixed salad leaves

Cook rice and lentils according to type, cool and add a variety of chopped vegetables such as pepper, cucumber, spring onions, celery, sweet corn, carrots, fennel, *anything you like* and stir in some olive oil, lemon/lime juice with a few nuts and seeds and selected fresh herbs (plenty of them) Or you could use spices mixed in a little olive oil (a curry paste).

Simple stir fry

One dessert spoon olive oil

Variety of vegetables i.e. broccoli, courgette/zucchini, peppers, mange tout (or sugar snap peas,) bean sprouts, carrots - anything you fancy or have in. Chopped or sliced.

Sauté/sweat a chopped onion and a clove of garlic. Add Grated ginger.

Add vegetables and cook to your liking, add a little water and some Tamari/soy sauce if liked.

Vary all the ingredients to create other tastes e.g. instead of ginger add mixed herbs, black olives.

Roasted Root Salad

This is delicious hot but also good when cold and/or eaten with rice, quinoa, millet or other grain.

2 lb parsnips, peeled and trimmed, cut into thick chips
1lb carrots, peeled and trimmed, cut into thick chips
4 Tbsp olive oil
14 oz cooked beetroot/beets peeled and chopped
One half an onion, finely diced
2 teaspoon chopped fresh herbs
Oven to 400 F/Gas 6/200 C electric

Place parsnips and carrots in a lightly oiled pan (using olive oil), then lightly brush them over with more olive oil plus a few tablespoons of water to prevent the vegetables drying out.

Cook for about 45 minutes turning halfway so that they get all crispy.

When cooked remove to a bowl and add the beetroot/beets, onion and herbs, mix and serve.

Quick Mixed Bean Chili - can be served with rice or other grain and a green salad

You can use tinned beans but ensure they are sugar free, drained and washed.

You can use carrots and carrot juice instead of tomatoes and tomato puree.

Sweat off 1 large onion and 2/3 cloves of garlic in a little olive oil add a pinch or more of chili powder, 1 tablespoon of tomato puree and paprika and cook for 1-2 minutes. Add tomatoes/carrots, beans and mixed vegetables (courgette/zucchini, carrots, peppers etc.) and cook until tender.

Quick Cashew Nut and Vegetable Pilaf - good hot or cold

Sauté 1 large onion and 2 to 3 cloves of garlic for about 5 minutes, add celery and peppers, brown rice 300g (1 ½ cups) uncooked weight, stir, add 1.5 pints (3 cups) of vegetable stock and bring to boil, turn down and simmer about 20 to 25 minutes until rice is cooked and liquid is absorbed. Stir in 4oz of chopped cashew nuts and some fresh parsley.

Vegetable Tikka

Choose vegetables to suit, ones that will cook easily or part cook before marinating. Chop, slice or cube courgette/zucchini, aubergine, sweet potato, peppers, tomatoes, fennel, mushrooms etc.

1 medium onion, 2 cloves, small piece ginger, 4 tablespoons soy yogurt or vegetable oil, juice of ½ lemon, 2 fresh chillies, 2 teaspoons coriander seeds, 1 teaspoon cumin, ½ teaspoon turmeric powder, fresh 10 mint leaves, ¼ teaspoon garam masala.

Dry roast seeds and grind, grind spices and add to rest of ingredients leave overnight or for several hours to marinate and then fast cook under grill or griddle until crispy

Serve with lemon and salad leaves and rice.

Penne Pasta & Red Pepper Sauce

1 large red pepper, and 1 onion for the sauce.

1lb rice pasta, 2 medium courgette/zucchini, 12 olives, 1 large onion, 2 cloves garlic, mixed fresh herbs (basil, marjoram, oregano,) 6 tablespoons olive oil, soft green peppercorns and squeeze of lemon juice.

Cook pasta in boiling water. In a separate pan sauté large onion (chopped, diced medium), courgette/zucchini, chopped garlic. Add all the ingredients to the cooked pasta and put into serving bowl.

For the sauce sauté the onions, add chopped peppers and ½ stock cube (yeast free). Cover with water, bring to boil and simmer for 30 minutes and either mix in with or pour over pasta dish.

Serve with large mixed salad.

Hummus

12oz chickpeas (soaked overnight), ¼ teaspoon ground cumin, 1 fresh chili, 1 clove garlic, 1 ½ tablespoons tahini, 4 tablespoons olive oil, 2 tablespoon lemon juice, pepper.

Boil the chickpeas approx 1-1.5 hours till tender then drain, saving a little of the water. Blend with other ingredients in blender or food processor till smooth. Add water if you want a thinner mix.

Salad Dressings

Oriental

6 tablespoons olive oil, 2 teaspoons of lemon juice, 4 teaspoons soy sauce, ½ teaspoon grated root ginger. Put into a jar and shake.

French

6 tablespoons olive oil, 2 tablespoons lemon juice, and 2 tablespoons cider vinegar. Variations on the above could include crushed garlic, balsamic vinegar, mustard and any fresh herbs you may like. Shake it all in a jar or put into a blender.

Soy Yogurt

Take a tub of natural soy yogurt and put in a blender with a choice of any herbs or spices, this will make a dressing or a dip for crudités. Whip in a blender.

Sun dried Tomato Dressing or Spicy if you add Chili

100ml (3 oz) olive oil, 2tablespoons tomato puree or sun dried tomatoes, 1 teaspoon each cumin, allspice, oregano, marjoram and a little cayenne pepper (vary any). Whizz in a blender.

Stuffed Peppers

4 peppers (1 for each person, reduce the whole recipe if just catering for one)

1 tbsp. olive oil

1 small onion finely chopped

1 clove garlic, minced

1 tsp. oregano

1 tsp. basil

2 carrots cut into fine sticks

1 Zucchini/courgette cut into fine sticks

1 tomato, diced

½ cup pine nuts or other nuts

1 ½ cups cooked wholegrain rice or quinoa

1 tbsp tomato puree

Preheat oven to 350 degrees gas 5/6

- Cut off tops of the peppers and remove seeds and membrane.
- Place on a suitable baking tray
- Heat oil in a frying pan or wok; add onion and garlic, sauté 1 minute.
- Add herbs, carrots and other vegetables
- Cook 3 to 5 minutes or until carrots are tender
- Reduce heat and add the tomato, pine nuts or other nuts, rice and tomato puree
- Stuff the mixture into peppers, don't worry if it overflows
- Bake in oven for 30 minutes or until peppers feel cooked to your liking

This can have a variety of vegetables or grains so make up your own stuffing and remember you can use this to stuff any stuffable vegetable. Try making a spicy one.

THE HEALTHY DUDE'S SUPER SHOPPING LIST

- o CHECK ALL LABELS TO ENSURE YOU ARE AVOIDING THE FOODS, ADDITIVES, INGREDIENTS THAT YOU ARE NOT SUPPOSED TO BE HAVING
- o BUY ORGANIC WHERE POSSIBLE
- o BUY WHAT IS IN SEASON AND LOCAL WHERE POSSIBLE

Store Cupboard Ingredient (Just a few ideas)

Rice Crackers, Oat Cakes, Corn Crackers

Porridge Oats, Millet, Quinoa *(pronounced "keen wa")*, buckwheat, Bulgur Wheat, Wholegrain rice *(basmati is good)*

Lentils, (green, red, brown) , Chick Peas, Mung beans, Black Turtle Beans, Black eyed beans, Kidney Beans, Flageolet Beans, Haricot Beans, Pinto Beans, Butter beans. *(All beans may be bought in tins but check no sugar/salt, cheaper and better to do your own from dried, see also sprouting.*

Yeast Free Stock Marigold Swiss Bouillon is good, low salt

Corn Flour, Rice Flour, Potato Flour, Soy Flour *(if you are going to do a lot of cooking/baking the different types of flour are useful)*

Rice Noodles, Rice pasta or corn pasta *(the latter minimal use)*

Herbs *(dried are ok but fresh where possible for better flavor)*

Spices *(will be dried in powder or seeds, use seeds where possible)*

Shitake and Porcini dried mushrooms

Tamari sauce, piri piri, balsamic vinegar, apple cider vinegar, Tahini. *(check those labels!)*

Extra Virgin Olive Oil, Canola Oil, Sesame Oil, Walnut Oil, Coconut Oil, Coconut Milk, Coconut Cream

Tinned Tomatoes (ok if fresh not available, check no sugar/salt.)

Sunflower, Pumpkin, Sesame, Flax/Linseeds - *don't forget you can sprout these!*

Black pepper, pure sea salt *(salt minimum use)* and mustard powder.

Fresh Ingredients, just a few ideas, buy what is in season and of course what you fancy

Fresh chillies, ginger, garlic

Fresh vegetables/salads and fruit, carrots, swede/rutabegas, turnips, parsnip, kohlrabi, sweet potato, squash/pumpkin, beetroot/beets, onions, garlic, scallions, shallots, artichokes, Cabbage red/green/white, spinach, kale, broccoli, brussels sprouts, cauliflower, asparagus. swiss chard, green beans.

Various herb leaves, lettuce, cucumber, courgette (zucchini), peppers, celery, aubergine/eggplant.

Tofu-in the refrigerated case (no flesh on the 30 day plan).

Lemons and Limes *(sliced added to hot water or for salad dressings)*

Hummus, Guacamole, *(check the ingredients as you could make your own quite easily)*

It's a good idea to keep a journal of the foods you eat on a daily basis. We have provided a template that you can download off my website and print on a weekly basis to track your intake. Go to www.TrishaStewart.com and head for the download section.

Chapter 4

Exercise

> *You see, you don't get old from age, you get old from inactivity, from not believing in something."* **Jack LaLanne**

Isn't age just a state of mind anyway? So, just because your driver's license states a certain age (and you really shouldn't lie about your age there) doesn't mean you have to let that number dictate how you feel or what you do. I realize most men don't worry about their age as much as so many women do, but I know you don't

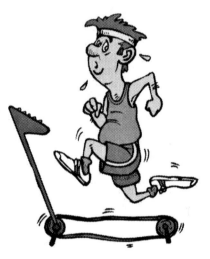

want to look any older than you have to. So, this chapter is all about *how to take you from Couch Potato to Healthy Dude!*

Okay, it's not going to come as any surprise to you that exercise is a vital part of living your best life and releasing your inner Healthy Dude. But, as a man...you actually have a leg up on working out. Typically, men are more likely to exercise to get it shape, rather than focus on what they're eating. In fact, a lot of men own up to working out so they can pig out (or at least eat what they want). So, I'm hoping you already understand some of the values of regular exercise (which by the way, isn't really so you can pig out). And, with the help of this book, my website – www.trishastewart.com – and Christin McDowell, the Trisha Stewart Team Fitness Guru and her book *Healthy Fitness Central*,, we'll show you the best way to get your "to die for" body.

Why bother working out?

Maybe you're not one of the men I mentioned above and exercise is something you avoid, detest or just don't see the value of at all. I have a friend that used to say, "Exercise is fascinating...I can watch other people do it all day!" Does that ring true for any of you? Well, just in case, I'm going to share some of the benefits of exercise. When combined with the correct diet, exercise can do amazing things for you besides helping you drop unwanted pounds, including: slow down the aging process, retard bone density loss and even lift depression. Here's a closer look at some of the battles regular exercise fights:

Cardiovascular and Respiratory Health/Heart Disease or Stroke

At best one of these could kill you off...but what would be worse is when they leave you severely disabled and not even able to hold down a job, be in a proper relationship or play with your kids and grandkids because part of your brain or body just doesn't work anymore... it's been too severely damaged. Yes, this is a reality; go visit the local hospital's cardio ward or maybe you already know someone who has had this happen to them. The heart is a muscle just like any other and needs exercise to keep fit. The more oxygen that flows through your lungs, the greater your cardio-respiratory (heart/lung) function. That's a good thing because the more clean air you take in the more waste is eliminated (through the lungs). And, the more oxygen you breathe in, the harder your heart has to pump for your muscles to receive the necessary oxygen and nutrients to work aerobically (aerobic means with oxygen). So, here are the benefits of aerobic exercise:

- Strengthening the muscles involved in respiration, to facilitate the flow of air in and out of the lungs.
- Strengthening and enlarging the heart muscle, to improve its pumping efficiency and reduce the resting heart rate.
- Toning muscles throughout the body.
- Improving circulation and reducing blood pressure.
- Increasing the total number of red blood cells in the body. Red blood cells transport oxygen.
- Reducing the potential for heart related problems.

Together with eating the right foods, exercise will help you to live a long and full on life.

Diabetes

While the main tools for avoiding diabetes are eating the right balance of foods and in the case of type 1 diabetes, insulin... Exercise is still a major part of actually preventing type 2 diabetes. If you already have this, managing it will be much easier when combined with the correct diet. People with diabetes are also encouraged to exercise regularly for better blood sugar control and to reduce the risk of cardiovascular disease. The reason for this is that working muscles use more glucose than those that are resting. Muscle movement leads to greater sugar uptake by muscle cells and lower blood sugar levels.

For those of you with type 1 diabetes, you may be able to reduce your insulin when working with a prescribed eating regime and program of exercises. But, check with your physician first and be very vigilant in testing your blood sugar levels. I believe that working with diet and exercise on a total prescriptive basis that some people can actually become insulin *independent*.

Type 2 diabetes can be reversed with a program of exercise and diet but this must be strictly adhered to because if your blood sugar has been out of control for sometime there may already be problems such as nerve damage. I have worked with people who have been diagnosed type 2 diabetes and seen a complete reversal. But, let me say that this is not easy work and is something you will always have to watch. Still, it becomes much easier once you have got the body's natural insulin doing its job properly.

Depression

It's about the endorphins...the happy hormones. When you exercise, your hormone system kicks in and releases endorphins, which lighten your mood and truly make you feel happier.

The word "Endorphin" comes from the two words, "endogenous + morphine." Endorphins are small, protein molecules that are produced by cells in your nervous system and other parts of your body. An important role of endorphins is to work with sedative receptors that are known to relieve common pain. These analgesia-producing receptors are located in your brain, spinal cord and other nerve endings. Endorphins are not a single molecule, but actually come in several forms, and can be anywhere from eighteen to five hundred times as powerful as any man-made analgesic. And, they are non-addictive into the bargain.

Endorphins have been shown to . . .

- Control persistent pain
- Control the craving for chocolate and potentially addictive substances

- Control feelings of stress and frustration
- Regulate the production of growth and sex hormones
- Reduce symptoms associated with eating disorders

You can see by these symptoms that exercise would combat a lot of the reasons behind depression...eating the wrong foods, not eating at all, stress and pain. I can promise you exercise will make you feel better, so make the time even if you really don't feel like it.

Bone Density, Muscles Tone and Connective Tissue problems

Muscles hold the skeleton in place, holding you up, holding you together and giving you good posture. Check the posture of others or even your own. Stand in front of the mirror. Are your knees bent? Is your belly sagging? Are you shoulders drooping? Are you even lopsided...one leg shorter than the other? This is lack of good muscle tone!

And, don't forget the connective tissue, ligaments and tendons...they are all an important part of "keeping it together". Ligaments are the fibrous, slightly stretchy connective tissues that hold one bone to another in the body, forming a joint. Ligaments control the range of motion of a joint, preventing your elbow from bending backwards, for example, and stabilizing the joint so that the bones move in the proper alignment.

While ligaments are slightly stretchy, they are arranged in crossing patterns to prevent the joint becoming loose. Stretching increases the length and flexibility of the muscles, allowing the joint to move farther than before. The ligaments themselves are not stretched, as they provide the support to the joint.

Tendons connect muscle to bone. The bones in a person's skeleton enable him or her to walk, run, jump, roll, lift, carry, drop, and do other important physical activities. Without the ability of tendons to connect the muscles and bones that are responsible for controlling these actions, it would be impossible for the body to move in the way it does. The ends of the muscles near the joints form into a more "bony" tissue, which are the tendons and they attach themselves to the bones.

Speaking of bones, participating in regular physical activity is probably the best thing you can do for them...especially when it is combined with good bone nutrition. And, here's a bit of trivia for you...physical activity during childhood and adolescence can potentially build bone mass that will still be with you as an adult. But that doesn't mean it's too late to help your bones. The right types of exercise also help to preserve bone strength into old age. So, as long as you can safely move, it is not too late to benefit from physical activity. I have just given you a peek at how the body is joined up, but remember...you have a marvelous body, keep it together.

More Benefits

There is a whole list of other concerns such as irritable bowel syndrome, fibromyalgia, headaches/migraines asthma, eczema that can be helped by exercise. Getting your body moving makes everything work better...including your organs. And, when you combine that with proper diet (you knew I'd have to mention that, right?), you've got everything you need to get into amazing shape. Plus, the difference in the way your clothes will hang on you is a major benefit! You may even find that you don't need to lose much weight after all...maybe your sagging belly was due to poor posture and lack of muscle tone. Check into chapter 7 for several additional therapies that will support your exercise journey (like massage and acupuncture). But, most important is to get yourself a personal trainer and sports therapist; they'll help create the perfect program for you needs.

Where is the best place to exercise?
The answer is anywhere you can make it work. Here are a few ideas to get you going:

- Run up and down the stairs at home or work
- Walk out the door and down the street, run or cycle anywhere there's a path or trail.
- Join a gym (or just go for the visitors pass – get in there)
- Running track (visit a local school during off hours)

- On the courts (tennis, basketball, racquet ball, volley ball...)
- On and in the water (swimming, skiing or walking along the shore)
- In the park
- On the snow
- On the skating rink
- On the golf course
- Up the mountains

Get it? Seriously, there's no excuse not to exercise. You don't have to own a fancy home gym, be a member of a fitness club or be a sports nut. You don't even have to leave your house...just walk the stairs, do some abdominal crunches, and see how far you can stretch your limbs...anything to get moving.

When is the best time to exercise?

How often should one exercise? Every day is the quick answer, but the type of exercise you do daily will depend on your age and fitness levels. If you're a bit older or more unfit, you need to be careful as you get started. Your best bet is to enlist the help of a professional. Of course, that's the way to ensure the best results at any age or fitness level which is why I have the very well qualified and experienced trainer Christin McDowell as a part of my team. She's here to help you 24/7 via the website- www.trishastewart.com

Two Types of Exercise

Aerobic training is any exercise that increases your heart rate and includes walking, cycling, running, swimming and racquet games and so on. Aerobic training is essential for the cardio vascular system and a typical session could be anywhere between 15-30 minutes, with a maximum heart rate of between 60-85 percent depending on age and fitness levels. Aerobic exercise can be, and should be done daily for maximum benefit.

Anaerobic training focuses on strength training such as weight training and should be two to three times weekly for about 30 - 60 minutes. Again, what you actually do depends on your age and fitness levels and the goals you want to achieve. If your vision is to be a body builder, or have the physique of one, you'll likely work out seven days a week, working different body parts each day. However, if your goal is just to be fit and lean – you won't need such intense workouts.

And please, a word to all you as you hit the gym or pick up the weights, don't just work your upper body. I've seen it too many times...men with amazing torsos and arms matched up with 'chicken legs'! So, get off the chest press and do a few deep squats! Remember, balance is the key to your best body.

How should you get started?

First of all, you'll do yourself a big favor if you get assessed for your fitness levels, factoring in your age and your goals. That's the best way to get started on the right track, doing exercises that are right for you. Remember everyone isn't ready to go out and run 10 miles, so be smart. On the other end of the spectrum, there are really no excuses to not do something! And, the excuses some people come up with run the gamut:

- I don't have the right shoes or any workout clothes
- I'm too busy with work, I don't have time
- I'm just too tired
- I can't get to the gym – it's not convenient
- I don't have room for a home gym
- I don't like the people who work out at my local gym
- I can't afford to work out
- My bike needs working on
- My skates are broken

But guess what? They're ALL EXCUSES...and all excuses are equal. So stop making them and start making yourself sweat instead!

Now certainly you can join a gym and that comes with pros and cons. It will cost you an annual membership, but you'll get an initial assessment and free use of the gym all day, everyday. The drawback is that after your first intro session where someone creates a program for you, you're on your own. You won't have anyone to show you what to do as your workout needs change. So please, I cannot stress this enough, keep an eye on your heart rate and maintain proper form. Don't assume you know what that is if you haven't worked out in a while, or if your body is changing as you lose weight and get in shape. The best solution is to work with a trainer, even if only periodically, to be sure you're always working out the right way. Remember, you can always visit the website, email Christin or get *Healthy Fitness Central* to get the right fitness support.

If joining a gym isn't your style, you cam buy some home equipment such as a multi-gym, rowing machine, stepper, cross trainer of elliptical trainer, barbells, dumbbells, fitness ball, inline skates, kayak, bicycle and so on. To figure out what type of equipment is right for you, define what you actually want to achieve. Perhaps you want to increase your cardio capacity, develop your core strength or improve flexibility...different equipment brings different benefits. And, very important, do you have the motivation to work by yourself. If the answer is yes, then find a good store (or reliable online shop) where you can talk through your needs to be sure you get the best equipment for your needs. Here's a quick run down of some home gym equipment:

Multi gym – this is, as the name says, a multi-exercise group of training equipment which you are pulling, pushing or lifting to train all body parts. They are relatively safe and take you through a full range of motion with good form and control. They isolate particular muscles or muscle groups which mean you can target areas that need working on with extra weights, and use lighter weights for those muscles that just need conditioning. Good for toning and strengthening muscles that have become wasted due to accident, injury or just lack of use.

Free weights – Barbells and dumbbells are great for home use because they can be stacked in a corner when you're not using them. But, they are dangerous if working alone. You can perform many different exercises using these weights and because they are what we call "free weights" you acquire better balance than when using a machine creating core stability. Form is essential here to ensure you do not injure yourself. So, take it slow and easy.

Rowing Machines - These will address body parts such as shoulders, abdomen and leg muscles so it is a good over-all piece of equipment. But, don't shop by price as cheap ones are a waste of money. They don't hold up to the amount of pulling and motion required for a good workout.

Treadmills - A good quality motorized machine will serve you well, especially if you have the model that elevates to mimic uphill walking or running. Certainly, this could be considered a luxury item, because you could just walk out your door and walk on the road or track. However, the benefits are low joint impact as opposed to road running, great aerobic activity that you can monitor, time saving as you don't have to leave the house and, of course, it's not dependant on the weather.

Cross/elliptical trainers – As with other larger machines, buy the best quality you can. It should offer a range of programs from weight loss to heart rate. The great thing about these machines is that they're low impact, which means gentle on the joints, feet and spine. You can burn quite a few calories, get a great cardiovascular workout and tone your legs and butt...all while watching TV or listening to your iPod. This is a great piece of equipment as long as you have the room...they can take up a bit of space.

Stationery bike - These are great for cardiovascular and leg tone. If you use it as a spinning bike, you can get an amazing workout (checkout further information on this great exercise if you're interested). Again, buy the best quality as it will provide you with a variety of exercises, plus last for years.

Fitness Ball - This is an amazing and inexpensive piece of equipment. It's fabulous for balance and core stability...just sitting on it works those muscles. But from sit ups to push ups it makes any exercise harder, because you have to keep still on the ball while doing the movements.

Outdoor equipment - If you don't have the space or interest in home gym equipment, getting some good outdoor equipment is a good option. Depending on your interests, you could buy a set of golf clubs, a tennis racquet, a kayak or a pair of roller blades. Whatever will inspire you to get outside and be active is what you should pursue. And, if you're not familiar with the sport or activity yourself, be sure you talk with someone who is an expert or plays to get advice on what to buy.

Okay, so we've talked about the benefits of exercise, how often you should exercise, how to get started, types of exercise and various types of equipment. We even talked about some of the excuses you might use to avoid exercise. So, let's take a look at some things to help keep you motivated to keep moving:

- Find someone that wants to compete with you or at least support you
- Set goals! Don't start out too big or you'll set yourself up for disappointment and failure. Don't plan to run a half marathon when you have never even trained for a sprint up the road
- Do something that you actually enjoy – so don't go to the gym weight training if you'd rather be playing tennis or another sport.
- Make it fun and enjoy the scenery... so while you're snowboarding or kayaking take a look around at what nature has to offer. Don't actually STOP and smell the roses (you need to keep moving), but do notice them as you jog by.
- Don't make it a mission – this can turn into mission impossible very soon.
- If you really can't make it one day – go the next, don't leave it for a week because it will just become harder.
- Find the schedule that works for you...shorter workouts more often may be better for you than 'marathon' sessions.

- Take a class to learn something new like yoga, Pilates or martial arts. You get great energy from being in a group, and there's built in accountability to show up!
- Keep a daily log – this will help you in moments of weakness. And, you may find you felt the same way a few weeks ago...but got through it.
- Schedule your workouts and put them into your day planner or calendar. If it's an appointment with yourself, you're more likely to do it. And, the more often you workout at the same time, the more it becomes second nature.
- Keep to around 30 – 60 minutes, depending on what kind of workout you are doing. Less won't give you the results you want and more begins to wear you down and you'll actually get less value.

Don't forget to exercise safely. I've already talked about using proper form and techniques, working with a trainer, taking classes and taking it slow. But there are a few other things to think about as a Healthy Dude is a safe dude!

- Stretch before you do anything at all – those muscles have been cramped up all day. Each muscle, including your heart, needs warming up so start with some gentle easy walking or running (even in place) and then slowly stretch out each muscle. Never bounce as you stretch and be careful not to push your muscles past a gentle stretch.

- Always wear the right clothing...to protect your body, help it breathe and sweat and to be sure you can be seen by others if you're on the road.

- Any water sport will require you wear a lifejacket, no matter how good a swimmer you are. Also for some water sports (like kayaking or white water rafting) crash helmets, knee protection and other body protection may be needed.

- Inline skaters wear knee and elbow pads plus a crash helmet.

- Cycling – off or on road - wear suitable clothing so you can be seen and please have some form of bell so that others know you are coming. Ever had a bicycle come right up behind you without you knowing! Crash helmets and gloves are a good bet too.

Some of you are ready to start your workout program right now. Others may want a bit more structure...and I've got that for you. Over the next few pages, Trisha Stewart Team's Certified Personal Trainer, Christin McDowell provides a look at three types of 'dudes' and the 'what to do' fitness steps to turn them into Healthy Dudes. So, figure out where you are now and what to do change. And, you can get additional help from the entire team at www.trishastewart.com. So, whether you're logging on for a more personalized program, heading out to join a gym or putting on your running shoes right now – just get moving. And, keep moving!!

The Healthy Dude Workout with Christin McDowell

"Being entirely honest with oneself is a good exercise."
Sigmund Freud

Men...you're lucky. Not only do you tend to prefer exercise over dieting (like Trisha mentions), but you get to eat more, naturally have less fat, have the hormones to make you less fat, you get to have more muscle and just about every organ in your body is bigger, better and stronger. 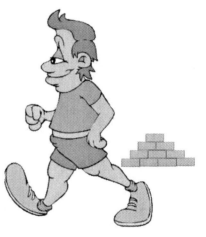 That doesn't mean you should shove twinkies and corn dogs into your face, but just be happy you don't have the struggle losing body fat that most women do. Now, with that said, there is no reason...I repeat...NO reason you should not be in shape. But, if you aren't in shape, don't worry. You've come to the right place to get yourself back on track.

Identifying Your Dude

Generally, I see three kinds of Dudes (besides the already Healthy Dudes and the super pumped 'Arnolds' of this world) out there:

- o **Dude #1 - You're really out of shape**
- o **Dude #2- You're kind of out shape**
- o **Dude #3- You just need a change in routine to lose the last "10" lbs (which, I've noticed with Dudes, is more like 30lbs).**

So, the first thing you need to do is identify which Dude best describes you. Go ahead, look in the mirror...who are you? Still not sure, I've got some basic descriptions below to help you see yourself and some things to focus on to help you get better results on your journey towards fitness.

Dude #1. You're really out of shape!

This looks like:

- You walk to the kitchen and call it exercise
- You walk upstairs to the bathroom and call it exercise
- You breath heavy after getting up off the couch
- Your pant size has seemed to move up 3-5 sizes in the past couple of years
- You make midnight runs for fast food or convenient store junk to get your quick fix "snack attack"
- You haven't literally tried to workout in years
- You life seems to be getting boring and people start ticking you off more and more

- Your heart hurts when you see those people and those people say things to you
- You haven't worked out in years

What you need to focus on

- Having the right Heart Rate
- The workout shouldn't be intense, but rather focus on the length and make your workouts longer before you make them more intense
- Pool workouts! (To give your joints and bones a break)

Dude #2. You're kind of out shape

This looks like:

- You have a gut, not a big one, but you got a gut
- You drink too much on the weekends and thus destroy any good habits you may have tried during the week
- Walking is somewhat difficult exercise
- You breathe really hard while watching Monday Night Football...even during the commercials
- You get winded walking up a flight of stairs
- You haven't worked out in months

What you need to focus on

- Committing to your workouts
- Committing to eating well, like a healthy dude would
- Not going buck wild on the weight training
- Not lifting so much weight you hurt yourself

- Wear good shoes because you need to start running for the first time in years
- Not drinking beer
- Not OD'ing on steaks
- Drink a lot of water

Dude #3. You just need a change in routine to lose the last "10" lbs (read 30lbs)
This looks like:

- Nice sized love handles that won't go away
- Can't see your six-pack abs
- Have had those very 10 lbs stay on you for a really long time...like maybe since high school (those pre-drinking years)
- You can do a pretty good job in your workouts, but need something to kick start the fire...to lose "the last 10lbs!"
- You work out about 3xwk

You need to focus on:

- Stop going wild on the weekends
- Change the way you workout
- Start adding sprints to your workout
- Start adding plyometrics to your workouts
- Do something physical you haven't done before...i.e. if you've never swam hard, swim hard!
- Get rid of the booze

- Start the 30 day detox plan in this book
- Workout about 4x/wk

Now What?

Okay, so now that you've figured out which "Dude" best describes you...what's the proper way to work out? I'm sure you've seen all the muscle and fitness magazines that come up with the new latest and greatest exercise. And, if you've tried any of those latest and greatest...you probably still look exactly the same. Here's what you need to know about workouts...there are three necessary steps for you to take:

1. Assess your Heart Rate
2. Come up with a 7 day layout Exercise Plan
3. COMMIT to your workouts

Assessing your Heart Rate

Assessing your Heart Rate is especially important for you #1's and #2 Dudes. If you're not already healthy and working out consistently, you want to steadily work up to the point where you are healthy and measuring your heart rate is a way of making sure you are not going too crazy your first months. This is the way to do it. If you have any kind of issue: high blood pressure, obesity, diabetes, etc. use this formula:

Heart Rate Reserve (HRR)

Target HR = (HR max −RHR) x.60 and .80 + RHR

(HR Max is always 220; RHR is Resting Heart Rate, See Below)

RHR means resting heart rate. You can count your pulse for six seconds add on a zero, or count it for 10 seconds and multiply by six.

If you don't have any issues or diseases, you can generally stick to THRZ:

220-(Your Age)= __x .6 = Low HR beats/min

220-(Your Age)= __x .85 = High HR beats/min

As you're starting your new workout, it's very important that you get a heart rate monitor so you can see where you're heart rate is throughout your workout. If your workouts feel too easy, then the range might be a little low. If you feel it's up too hard, then the range is probably too high. Your body is the best judge. However, if you fit in the HRR category, your exercise might feel easy but your heart rate range is right where it should be. Because of this, focus on having longer workouts instead of harder workouts.

After about two - three months of working out (four times a week), you will notice your cardiovascular fitness improving and therefore you should reassess where your heart rate should be. And yes, one day, you won't have to use the heart rate monitor anymore! Until then, monitor your heart rate and check with your doctor to see if it's a good range for you!

Come up with a 7 Day Layout

Being the busy men you are, you need to have a plan to make sure you have workout time scheduled. So, make a plan. Choose certain days of the week you are sure you can fit your workouts in, schedule the time on your calendar and do it!! Remember not to prioritize money over your health...it's not worth it. Choose those days and stick to them like gum on the bottom of your shoe! Here is an example of what a 7 day schedule should look like:

Monday	Tuesday	Wednesday	Thursday	Friday	Saturday	Sunday
CV 45-50 Min	CV 5-10Min WRKT weights #1	OFF or LT Pool wrkt	CV 45-50+ Min	CV 5-10 Min WRKT #1	OFF	Pool

(CV: Cardiovascular Work, LT: Light, WRKT: Workout)

Commit to your Workouts

The change in your body will happen, but it'll take a little time. You didn't just gain 30 pounds overnight, so you won't be able to get rid of it in two weeks. It's important you commit yourself to your goals and remember you need to be persistent in order to see results. It will happen if you do it, so stick with it and commit to it. And, by following the 30 day plan you are virtually guaranteed to lose weight, especially if you exercise too.

If you don't see results as soon as you'd like them...DON'T STOP!! Just re-evaluate what you're doing because you are probably doing something wrong. It could be the duration of your workouts or the type of exercise. But, chances are it's what you're eating though and not your workouts. In other words...eating too much or the wrong types of food. Thankfully this whole book is dedicated to making sure you are eating right, so follow it!

Ok, so how do I structure my workouts?
It all depends on your level of fitness and what your goal is. What you really need to do is check out *Healthy Fitness Central*, where I have in-depth tailored workouts and layouts for men for all fitness levels, body types and goals. You have to train differently if you have different amounts of muscle mass, if you have pre-existing conditions such as high blood pressure and obviously to train for your goal. With that said, here are some things Dude #1, #2, #3 needs to focus on with their workouts:

Dude #1
Because your body is in a "sick" mode right now, (high blood pressure, high body fat) you'll need to have an easier program that focuses on cardiovascular training and very little weight training. The last thing you want to do is a bunch of heavy weight lifting, as it could push your already high blood pressure even higher causing further damage to your body.

A good program would be cardio within your heart rate_4-6x/wk, 45-60 min. If you feel like doing more or less, it's important you listen to your body and progress only when it's telling you to. Don't do too much too soon, but make sure you are doing enough. As you progress you'll get better at listening to and being in tune with your body, but I think it's best you run your program by your doctor or naturopath for a qualified 'okay' on your workout.

As far as weight training, you should stick to using your own body weight right now. These would include:

- Push ups on your knees- exhaling as you press up
- Abdominal Crunches
- Step Ups
- High knees
- Butt kicks

All these exercises are shown on the website and in Healthy Fitness Central

*Always make sure you are breathing through your exercises.

The reason I like to have you do your own body weight in the first few months is because chances are you're already carrying around 50+ pounds all day long with your extra body weight, so why add on more??? Your muscles already work hard enough as it is, so it's better to focus on burning body fat, increasing your cardiovascular capacity and getting in shape. Leave the weight training until after you've dropped about 20-25 pounds. You can then move on to Dude #2's workout when you feel ready. *Please refer to Healthy Fitness Central for detailed timelines and programs.

Dude #2

So just like Dude #1, you need to get your base line cardiovascular fitness down. If you have not committed to a fitness program in the past, do it now! You'll also need to wear a heart rate monitor at least for the first three months. Your basic workout should include 4-5x/wk cardio and 2x/wk body weight exercises with light to moderate weight training. You can do your cardio on the same day as your weights. *I would start weight training only after about 1 month of getting your cardiovascular fitness up.*

Layout

Monday	Tuesday	Wednesday	Thursday	Friday	Saturday
CV 25 Min Weights/Body wt Rx 5 min SS Cardio	CV 45-60min	OFF or Pool	CV 25 Min Weights/Body wt Rx 5 min SS Cardio	CV 45-60m	OFF

CV: Cardiovascular work: Running, Elliptical, Pool. NOT sitting down on the stationary bike the entire time!

Wt Rx: Weight training exercises 12-15 Reps, Breath! Light-Moderate Weight

- Seated Back Row
- Chest Press
- Military Press, Shoulder Raise
- Curls

SS: Super Set (1 exercise directly followed by another)

Body WT RX: Body weight exercises- 10-20 Reps

- Push ups
- Full sit ups
- Butt lifts
- Squats
- Step ups
- Plank Hold
- Up Up Down Downs

Then, after your one month of Cardiovascular Training, you can start doing the following workout:

- CV 25 Min
- Weights/Body wt Rx 5 min
- SS Cardio

This means, after you do 25 minutes of cardio (anything but a stationary bike), do a round of body weight or weight training exercises followed by two minutes or so on the elliptical or running if you can. Then repeat the weight training and two minutes of cardio until you've done three to four rounds. You can then cool down by walking for a few minutes until your heart rate goes down. After you've done a few months of this, progress on to the next level which you will find in Healthy Fitness Central.

Dude #3

So you've put in a lot of hard work, a lot of liters of sweat; Maybe turned down some cold beers and yet your belly still isn't showing it's beautiful six-pack. You're getting frustrated and are willing to accept that you'll always have that extra weight or that spare tire. Wrong! You can and will lose that fat if you want to; it's all up to you. The first step you need to do is evaluate your training program. You need to start doing things you've never done before. Your system needs something to stimulate it and to kick start it's metabolism, which if you read on I'll tell you how to do.

Are you following the plan in this book ? That means sticking with it, not just through the week, but on the weekends too. That way every Saturday and Sunday you don't undo all the good you did the previous week. You really must work at this, if it was easy, everybody would be doing it, you are special so make sure you treat yourself that way.

Kick Start Training

Some of the best training tactics I've seen men respond to are anaerobic training and super setting exercises with plyometrics. Anerobic training literally means without air-oxygen. An example would be an all out 100% sprint for 50meters or during a wrestling or swim match. There are many reasons why anaerobic training is so effective.

- Your cardiovascular system has to work hard to recover which means that your resting heart rate, blood pressure, and recovery time are all going to improve faster
- You will have a greater ability to burn fat for the prime energy source at a higher intensity
- You will become faster and stronger-with more developed "Type A" muscle fibers
- Your testosterone levels respond well to this form of training, which means more body fat loss and greater muscular response

Plyometrics are anaerobic and consist of exercises such as jumps and fast movements which stimulate the nervous and muscular-skeletal system in a huge way. They can be done after larger more powerful movements such as the squat or chest press. Plyometrics have all the positive responses you see with anaerobic movements, as they are anaerobic.

An example of this would be:

- One set Mod/Heavy Squat , Reps of 4-6, directly followed by a set of Squat Jumps 8-10 Reps
- One Set of Heavy/mod Chest Press directly followed by Push Up Claps x8

In Healthy Fitness Central there are 2 whole workouts that are designed with plyometrics and anaerobic training under "Super Jock". Follow this workout and see your body change!

Training Layout

You should be working out at least 4x/week. I would recommend two days with a lot of anaerobic training followed either by a rest day or a lighter intensity day. This will allow your body to heal and increase its performance capacity. Pool workouts are awesome for you because of the effect they have on your cardiovascular system. They also have no impact on your muscles and bones after an intense day of anaerobic training. Days where you want to just do some simple cardio or biceps are good too and should be included when your body is ready.

An example Program would look like this:

Monday	Tuesday	Wednesday	Thursday	Friday	Saturday	Sunday
Anaerobic Workout	Swim 50min	OFF	Anaerobic Workout	Aux/CV	OFF	Pool or OFF

AUX: Auxiliary training (limb lifts; biceps curl, quadriceps ext, hamstring curl, etc)

So, if you want to get in the best shape of your life and lose the last 10 pounds, it's not too late! You're never too old to get in awesome shape and start looking good. Try some of these training tactics and if you are ready, read more in Healthy Fitness Central. Healthy Fitness Central has all the programs, exercises and pictures you need to be well on your way to having the best Healthy Dude body around!

Chapter 5

Inside the Healthy Dude

Your emotions affect every cell in your body. Mind and body, mental and physical, are intertwined. - ***Thomas Tutko***

Ever wonder why sometimes when you're nervous or anxious you get an upset stomach? Why does stress result in tight muscles (especially the neck and shoulders)? The answer is because everything you feel and experience manifests itself in your body. In other words how you feel emotionally 'shows' in how you feel physically. And those feelings can also affect choices you make. You've had a bad day and you're 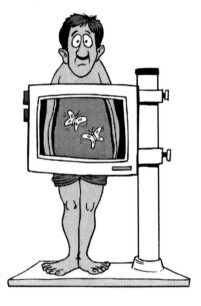 really tired, so instead of going for a run, you grab a beer and watch television. I know 'you've' never done that before, but you get the idea, right? I'm a strong believer in mind-body connection, but I've got some good news...this chapter *ISN'T about your feelings!*

Still, there's more to being a Healthy Dude than what you look like on the outside, right? And, while eating right and exercising (as I've laid out in Chapters 3 & 4) are the basis for your new healthy lifestyle, you really need to have an understanding about what's going on inside your body. That way you'll have a clue if something isn't going right. So, while we won't get into examining your feelings (I know – WHEW!), we will take a look at how you feel on the inside, why and what you can do about it to make things better.

Digestive Problems

You know I've already laid out how the digestive system works in Healthy Dude Eating (chapter 3), but it's a little more complex that what goes in eventually comes out. What I haven't shared with you is some of the digestive challenges you may be trying to cope with on your own. In fact, you may have some problems you don't even realize are connected to your digestion. So, here's a more in-depth look at some digestive woes you may be suffering from too frequently:

- Bloating – That feeling of being full but hungry, rumblings going on and loads of gas...and it feels as if your gut is stretched to the max.
- Constipation – This can go on for days or more. People tell of hard and dry stools, not feeling fully evacuated, passing water and this feeling of complete discomfort. Believe it or not, 'back in the day' people occasionally

died of constipation (they didn't know how to treat it...but today, luckily, we do!).

- Diarrhea - This can have you rushing to the toilet ten times daily or just once a day, but whenever you go, you pass a very loose motion. The colon and anal passage can become inflamed and potentially cause fissures in the rectum. That means major discomfort and pain.

- Colitis - A very aggressive form of diarrhea, Colitis often accompanies blood, this is not a good thing to have as it can lead to ulcerative colitis and eventually cancer. Symptoms are similar to extreme diarrhea but the associated pain is far worse. The sufferer cannot leave the house at times or if they do they need to know every public toilet on route. Being at work can be very difficult. Dehydration and lack of nutrition can be very weakening to the person.

- Alternating constipation and diarrhea - or good old IBS (irritable bowel syndrome) as the doctors have named it.

Well, those all sound like fun, don't they? Everyone has a problem now and then...you eat something that doesn't agree with you, get the stomach flu, or have problems when you travel. That's not what I'm talking about here. What I'm talking about is ongoing problems that you're dealing with on a weekly, maybe even daily basis. No one should have digestive problems every day. If you do, no matter which one of the above (or combination), guess what - they all have some things in common:

- Poor diet
- Sometimes poor hygiene including food poisoning
- Stress (this will cause the gut to become compromised)

But wait...there's more!!! Yes, there are a few more ailments that could be bothering you (or may soon if you're not living the Healthy Dude way).

- Diverticulitis - Diverticuli are small protrusions in the wall of the colon almost like a hernia, if they become inflamed they bleed and cause cramping and pain in the abdomen and bouts of constipation/diarrhea.
- Ulcers - These can be anywhere along the digestive track but are usually in the duodenum, which is part of the stomach - they may bleed and cause extreme pain.
- Over acidity - When the upper gastric (from stomach up to mouth) seems to be inflamed and very painful. It's that awful burning sensation that makes you swear your insides are on fire.
- Indigestion - Similar to above
- Heartburn - Similar to above
- Parasites - No one usually knows they have these bacteria but they can cause havoc...then you KNOW you've got them! Apart from digestive problems these can cause fatigue and symptoms associated with Candida.

- Candida – This is so common. It's one of the normal bacteria that live in our bowel - one of the bad guys - but if it is allowed to grow it will cause a myriad of symptoms and is known as candidiasis (see chapter 6 and my website for more on this).

- Crohn's disease – Similar symptoms to above but also includes weight loss, fatigue, fever and is much like having food poisoning on a regular basis. I have found those diagnosed with this problem to have one or more of the above symptoms and can be helped if not cured. Crohn's affects more men than women and at quite an early age. And, here's something to note - if you get a diagnosis from your doctor, it ends up in your medical file and can actually lead to problems with insurance and possible career moves. So, before you go to your regular GP, seek alternative help where possible and like every disorder, the sooner you get it checked the easier it will be to deal with.

- Colon cancer – When all or some of the above get out of hand, the result is often cancer. But, there are early warning signs of all these issues and they can be dealt with and treated...so do it! Don't ignore any ongoing digestive issues!

And guess what – I know this may not surprise most of you that I'll say this - like the first few maladies, these are also linked to poor diet and stress. I have seen all of these cases in my clinic and helped every one of them who have had these diseases and symptoms with great success – all through changing the diet! So, this isn't just something I'm saying to convince you to eat differently...it's proven to work!

Skin Conditions

Okay, you're probably thinking, 'Trisha – my skin is on the outside of my body - I thought we were looking at what's going on inside.' Well, you're right, except that with the skin we see the end result of the problems on the outside, but it's almost always something going on internally that causes that problem in the first place. So, let's take a quick look at some of the most common skin conditions.

Eczema

Eczema covers a broad range of skin conditions akin to dermatitis where the upper layers of skin become inflamed. This can be accompanied by dryness, skin rashes, redness, swelling, itchiness, flaking and crusting, blisters, cracking between the fingers, oozing and even bleeding. But, there are different types of eczema, with different symptoms and causes:

1. Atopic – Sometimes called hereditary, Atopic can run in families. Sufferers also often have hay fever and asthma – the body is producing histamines to an allergic response of some kind. It may also be linked to stress

and the nervous system. Atopic eczema can be cured by natural medicine and diet.

2. Contact dermatitis - This looks very similar to Atopic and is definitely an allergic response to a chemical or plant. It too, can be treated with natural medicine and diet as together these improve the whole body response to anything that may irritate it.

3. Xerotic - People who suffer from very dry and cracked skin can develop this. It usually appears during the winter or summer months...or extreme temperatures... accompanied with the individual becoming dehydrated. The condition resembles that of a dry riverbed, with the skin all cracked and dry. The best treatment for Xertoic eczema is to ensure you are massively hydrated with pure water, not tea, coffee or soda and find a natural hydrating cream that will help to heal the cracks.

4. Seborrheic dermatitis - This is often found around the scalp and eyebrows can be dry or greasy and cause red patches to appear. In newborn babies it is called cradle cap and can be linked to a biotin deficiency. In adults this can be the same, a diet related issue. Therefore adjusting the diet (i.e. adding back in the missing nutrient) takes care of it.

5. Dyshidrosis - Can you believe this is sometimes called housewife's eczema?? I know - very sexist! But, that doesn't mean men can't get it as well. It occurs on the

palms of hands and the sides of the fingers, soles of the feet and toes. It starts off as tiny blister like bumps and then thickening of the skin, cracks and of course itching which is worse at night and in warm weather. Although there is no one specific cause, it seems to be aggravated by prolonged exposure to the sun, exposure to chlorinated or highly treated water, some soaps and cleaners (hence the awful nickname). Keeping skin dry will speed the healing.

6. Venous – This condition shows up on people with poor circulation, varicose veins and edema (fluid retention) around the ankle area. It's most common in people over the age of 60 and symptoms are areas of skin that redden, darken and itch. Leg ulcers can also occur. If exercise is not possible, when sitting, raise the legs on a stool, to be above the waistline so the fluids drain away from the infected areas. Specific massage and drainage techniques will also improve this. See chapter 7.

7. Dermatitis herpetiformis –This is directly linked to celiac disease, but diagnoses of celiac (an extreme allergy to gluten) is difficult. It typically occurs as a rash on arms, thighs, backs of knees and back, but can be more widespread due to individual severity. A corrective diet (gluten-free) will treat the symptom, but it can take months for the skin to clear.

8. Neurodermatitis – Most often caused by stress, this form of eczema is usually one spot on the body where the skin thickens and the pigment changes due to habitual rubbing.

9. Autoeczematization – Unlike many skin conditions, this is usually a reaction to parasite, fungi, bacteria or viruses. The trick to curing this is to find the specific cause and addressing/eliminating the source.

Okay, so you've probably just learned more about eczema than you ever wanted to, but it's important you understand that all 'itchy skin' is not the same. That being said, if you have any rashes, blisters or outbreaks that don't seem normal, you really should get them checked out as soon as possible. Knowing what's going on is half way to the cure!

Psoriases

Many people lump eczema and psoriases into the same category, but they have quite different symptoms. This awful condition can affect the joints and the skin and causes red patches to appear on the skin which become scaly and raised. As it's related to the joints, it typically affects the knees, elbows but also the scalp, but it's not unheard of in severe cases for the entire body to be affected. Finger and toe nails can be affected and when they are, it causes a yellowing of the nail, thickening of the skin underneath the nail, as well as a loosening and crumbling of the nail. This is a recurring condition which varies in severity from the proportion of the body that it is affecting and the degree of redness and plaque occurring at these sites. There are different forms of psoriases that include:

- **Plaque psoriases** - The most common form of psoriases, appearing as raised areas of inflamed skin covered with a white scaly skin.
- **Flexural** - This type is most often found around the genital area, under the breast or stomachs of an overweight person. These appear as smooth inflamed patches and due to the areas these are in can be prone to fungal infections.
- **Guttate** – Guttate consists of lots of small spots over the body and sometimes scalp. It's often associated with a viral condition.
- **Pustular** – This form of psoriases can appear anywhere on the body and is indicated by raised bumps that are full of pus with the surrounding skin quite red and tender.
- **Psoriatic** – Psoriatic psoriases involves swelling of the joint and connective tissue and most commonly occurs in the finger and toe joints.
- **Erythrodermic** – This may be the most dangerous type of psoriases. It is characterized by widespread inflammation, excessive exfoliation, severe itching, swelling and extreme pain. It's dangerous because it

affects the body's ability to regulate temperature...and that can be fatal. Remember, your skin acts as a barrier or protective shield for your body and regulating your temperature is a part of that protection.

I have seen all of types of psoriases in my clinic and I always start with correcting and working with balancing the diet. So, clearly that's step one. I'm not saying you should self-diagnose...that's not a smart idea. But, before you pump your body with antibiotics, steroids and whatever else one might attempt to treat the symptoms...look first to the cause! I promise you a healthier diet will make a difference! Stress is a major factor here too, so lifestyle coaching is a great idea or go to chapter 7 and investigate natural ways to eliminate stress.

Fungal Infections

Hmmmm...this doesn't seem like a very fun topic, but then neither is eczema or psoriases, right? But, once again, this is stuff you need to know. Fungal infections can happen anywhere and, are a lot more common than you might think. They can develop in any orifice, crevice, fold of skin or on your scalp, hair and nails. Seriously...think about mushrooms...where do they grow? They flourish in damp, warm and dark conditions. Well, guess what...mushrooms are fungi! Don't panic, I'm not saying if you don't wash between your toes you'll start growing mushrooms...but I am saying you cannot be too diligent about being sure you're clean and dry!! So, let's talk about fungi!

First, since I've been talking about skin conditions, we'll start with fungal skin infections.

Fungal Skin Infections

Fungal skin infections can be rashes or red scaly and itchy patches in the hair, on the scalp, in folds of skin and on finger or toe nails. The infections can often be confused with eczema or other skin conditions, but their cause is very different. Here's a look at some types of fungal infections:

- *Athlete's foot (Tinea Pedis)* – Probably one of the most common, because even if you've never had it; you've heard of it. It's typically found between the toes, the skin is "soggy" itchy and becomes infected with bacteria very easily. It's passed from human to human by skin droppings in public places such as swimming pools and locker rooms. It can be very contagious in some individuals. Hint: Wear shower shoes at the pool or in the gym locker room!
- *Nail infections (Onychomycosis or Tinea Unguim)* - This is ringworm of the nails, and is actually fairly common. The nails become thickened, discolored and crumbly. It occurs when the nail plate is separated from the nail bed...and there's room for fungus to grow. The conditions are things like tight footwear and communal showers (moist and dark, remember?)

- *Jock Itch (Tinea Cruris)* – This one men don't like to talk about too much, but it can affect many athletes or sports enthusiasts due to sweating causing damp and heat in the groin area. And, it can be 'two for the price of one' because it often accompanies athlete's foot as scratching one area can lead to passing it to the other. I'm not saying you guys are always scratching yourselves, but...

- *Ringworm (Tinea Corporis)* – Usually, this is called ringworm and can be found in patches anywhere on the body. It appears as a scaly edge with clear skin in the center and can be contracted from domestic animals.

- *Scalp Ringworm (Tinea Capitas)* – Most often ringworm of the scalp affects young children and can cause hair loss. It's spread by contact with another who has it or by someone who may not even have the symptoms but is a carrier. A little tricky, isn't it? Again, stay clean and dry!!

What makes you more susceptible to exterior fungal infections?
- Taking antibiotics
- Oral steroids (including inhalers)
- Diabetes
- Obesity
- Weakened immune system
- Moist skin after sweating
- Open wounds

Candida Albicans

Although this is also a fungal infection, it's such a massive topic and issue; I'm going to spend some extra time on this. And, keep in mind; I'm just scratching the surface on this one. Basically Candida is one of the normal bacteria that reside in our digestive system and mouth. But, it's one of the "bad guys" and like a weed it can overrule the garden and become a pest. When this happens, it's called candidiasis. Candida (and other yeast) lives in us all, mostly without causing any harm. But, when the diet includes a lot of sugar and yeast, Candida feeds off of it, grows and overrides the growth of good bacteria. This is when it can row into its fungal form and spores permeate through the intestinal wall into the rest of the body. The medical profession does not accept this as a problem in general making it very difficult to get a medical diagnosis of Candida, yet they diagnose thrush!

However, it can be a major problem for some people; I've seen countless clients with it. So, I'm going to go over the symptoms and contributing factors.

Common symptoms of Candida

Okay, even if you do accept that too much Candida is a problem, it can still be difficult to diagnose. That's because some sufferers have numerous symptoms and others may only have some minor ones. And, even if you have symptoms...those symptoms could be related to a different condition. So, please don't read this list and think "I have got all of these it must be Candida." While you need to be aware of what's going on with your body, don't guess what you may or may not have...get it checked out to be sure. Leaky gut syndrome, caused by Candida and parasites often leads to:

- Food allergies and intolerance
- Migraines/headaches
- Foggy brain
- Muscle aches
- Thrush
- Joint pains
- Asthma
- Hay fever
- Sinusitis
- Fungal infections of the nails/skin e.g. athlete's foot
- Ear infections
- Chronic tiredness
- Allergies
- Sensitivity to perfume, tobacco smoke and petrol
- Bloatedness
- Flatulence
- Diarrhea and/or constipation
- Itchy anus
- Weight gain or weight loss

Candida has also been implicated in ME and CFS (Myalgic Encephalomyelitis, Chronic Fatigue Syndrome), Fibromyalgia and other immune diseases.

Contributory Factors

So, what are you taking, using or being exposed to that could increase your chances of having a problem with Candida? Take a look:

- Use of antibiotics
- Use of other steroids (hydrocortisone, prednisone etc.)
- Use of immuno-suppressive drugs
- repeated use of broad-spectrum antibiotics e.g. for acne
- Dental mercury amalgam poisoning
- Other heavy metal poisoning e.g. lead, cadmium
- Chemical poisoning from the home, garden, workplace etc.
- Hormonal changes e.g. puberty, pregnancy, menopause
- Stress

For any type of fungal infection prevention is, obviously, your first choice. And, as I've said throughout the previous pages...that's about staying clean and dry and just being aware of what's going on with your body. But, if you already have a fungal infection, then you have to deal with treatment...and be patient. A combination of diet (especially in dealing with Candida), topical lotions and creams can all play a great part in relief and healing. But it can take quite some time to clear up. That means regular application of ointments; diligent eating habits and ongoing good hygiene...real patience! Again, I've dealt with almost every one of these issues in my clinic, so I have answers for you. If you're dealing with Candida or another fungal infection...or you're not sure what you're dealing with, please visit my website at www.trishastewart.com to get a detailed treatment plan for your specific needs.

Asthma

Okay...away from the skin, no more talk about fungi! Let's talk about your breath...or to be more specific, your breathing and a condition called asthma. This respiratory system ailment used to be rare, but these days it's becoming so very common. It seems more and more people are being diagnosed with asthma.

I feel this is due to some of the following:

- Pollution and poor air quality
- Use of aerosols, deodorants, hair spray etc
- Cosmetics
- Shampoo
- Sun cream
- Hair gel
- Toxic house cleaning materials and the aerosols they are often contained in
- Paints and other decorating materials
- Tobacco and smoke fumes

- Animal dander
- Dust mites
- Chlorine at the swimming baths
- Perfumes and aftershaves
- Stress
- Puberty and hormonal changes

What happens with asthma is this...the airways to the lungs, which are called bronchials, become constricted or narrowed, inflamed and lined with an excess mucus. This happens in a response to the allergen affecting the individual, and the result is wheezing, shortness of breath, coughing, increased heart rate, the inability to exhale (which is the most frightening), chest tightness and the chest expanding. And, in severe cases, people can turn blue through lack of oxygen and collapse. How often these 'attacks' happen varies from person to person. For some it's only occasional breathing difficulties, but for others it's literally a daily episode...especially if they've become hypersensitive to allergens.

What can be done?
If you (or someone you live or work with) is dealing with asthma, there are some things that can improve their situation. First of all, get rid of all the chemical laden cleaning materials, deodorants, paints and all the things I have listed above. There is no need for any of it; they can all be replaced with eco-friendly products. If you can't find natural products at a local

store – hit the Internet where there are lots of sites you can shop. And, get a peak flow monitor...that way you can check regularly to see what improvements have been made since clearing out chemicals. Next, you must start exercising! Work with a personal trainer who understands respiratory conditions and what you can and cannot do.

Sometimes you just need to "blow" the airways. Using seed oils can help with inflammation, as will physiotherapy, air ionizers, acupuncture, chest tapping and vibration, posture, yoga, Pilates and more. And, you may need to examine where you live. Do you live in a damp house, near water or lots of trees? That could be a contributing factor to your asthma...so if all else fails, you might consider moving to a different neighborhood or climate. All of these things will help asthma sufferers, but it's only part of the whole program.

Diet! That's right...I bet you wondered when I would get around to this one, didn't you? I have helped and dare I say, even cured, people with asthma just through changing their diet; I focus on taking out all the foods that encourage mucus to build. That's why removing dairy and wheat are two of the most important dietary choices to make in this case. Of course, there are also many preventative products available by prescription, and I'm not saying you shouldn't use something for those major asthma attacks while you're getting your condition under control. But, those medicines have some serious side effects. Inhalers are just steroids taken orally and they can cause a hoarse voice or oral thrush. And corticosteroids cause a redistribution of fat, increased appetite, blood glucose problems, weight gain and osteoporosis. So, please always try the natural route, you have nothing to lose.

Depression

Let me quickly say that in this book I am NOT addressing clinical depression or bi-polar disorder. Those are other subjects entirely and require very special care. The type of depression I'm going to address is a state of mind...stronger than a mood...caused by a series of events.

Let's face it; we all get a bit fed up from time to time. Things don't go quite how we would like them to go (or nothing like we'd like them to go)...the weather is not good... the job is boring...the person we love leaves us (or makes it difficult to love them)...lots of little triggers can end up making us feel absolutely miserable. This awful feeling may last for a day or perhaps a couple of weeks – but it passes. It always passes, eventually...right? Well, it should. But, take a look at the list below. If six or less of these symptoms apply to you, then chances are you're just fed up...you need a change in lifestyle, or environment. A day off from work (especially if you played hooky) would do you wonders! But, if more than six of these symptoms describe you, then chances are you have had a form of depression for a while and it's not going to just 'pass' on its own.

So, how many of these statements describe you:

- Feeling unhappy – most of the day, but improve late in the day.
- Feel worse at a particular time each day
- Lose interest in general life
- Can't seem to find enjoyment from anything that you used to enjoy
- Find it hard to look for anything that you would find enjoyment from
- Tired all the time
- Loss of confidence and feeling of being inadequate
- Can't get to sleep, taking one or more hours
- Lack of interest in sex or loss of libido
- Weight loss or weight gain
- Anxious and restless
- Irritable
- Can't make normal day to day decisions
- Avoid meeting others socially or in the street

As I said, we've likely all experienced some or most of these at a time or two in our lives. But, if you find yourself facing six or more of these 'characteristics' then chances are you've felt this way for far too long. But there IS something you can do about it. First, please don't blame yourself. People often feel if they were 'stronger' they could 'get over it'. Well, losing a loved one, retiring, being unable to find suitable employment or losing a job are all things that can make you feel depressed. The other reaction is to blame someone else...the person who died, who left you, who fired you, who didn't hire you...whatever. That's normal, but they're really not the cause of your depression.

If your immune system has become compromised during or after illness, this can leave you feeling low – it can be confused with depression.

I always say 'mind invades body'...in this case while being sick won't make you depressed (although a compromised immune system can leave you feeling temporarily low), being depressed can trigger health issues like headaches, nausea, sleeplessness and irritable bowel. So, besides not blaming yourself or others...what can you do about depression?

- Talk to a friend or family member that you can trust (it is NOT a sign of weakness to talk about how you're feeling. It's often the first step to feeling better)
- Go outside for a walk or do some exercise on a regular basis (even if you don't feel like it...push yourself!)
- Get a life coach or counselor - seek out a therapist who specializes in depression (see chapter 7 for more details on that); seek out why or if you are depressed or just fed up.

- Rest, even if you don't sleep, use some relaxation CDs or guided meditation
- Diet – you knew I'd say that...but I say it only because it's true!

  1. Cut out all stimulants, coffee, tea, alcohol, cigarettes, drugs - these will only serve to lift you for a short space of time, but drop you deeper into depression when not using them, they will become addictive, if not already.

  2. Stop adding sugar to drinks – this will raise the blood sugar giving you a feeling of energy, only again to drop you further down the hole.

  3. Stop eating cakes and cookies, chocolate, puddings, ice cream and other sweets for the same reason.

  4. Ditch the soft drinks – full of chemicals and sugar

  5. Start to eat slow release carbohydrates and plenty of vegetables and salads. Follow my 30-day detox plan (chapter 3) and you'll be amazed how you feel afterwards.

  6. Try to do without anti-depressants, if you are already taking them talk to a professional about coming off them and take natural alternatives.

Depression is a serious matter and there's plenty of help available so you don't have to go through your days feeling bad, sad and just plain awful. So, talk to someone, try my recommendations and don't go it alone.

Headaches/Migraine

You've had a headache...I'm sure of it. In fact, I'd be quite shocked if you could say to me you never had one. But a migraine is a different animal...not everyone suffers from them and if you don't, it's hard to understand how excruciating they can feel. So let's take a look at both of them.

A headache can be something that comes on for a variety of reasons...working in an office with powerful lighting, poor eyesight or incorrect eye glasses, too much time at a computer, dehydration and stress. They can actually come and go in a matter of a few hours or less...often without any treatment (if you can put up with the pain for a bit).

A migraine can certainly be triggered by all of the above but also an allergen such as perfume, chemicals, pollen, pollution and poor diet, hormonal changes and postural problems - particularly upper spine and neck. The pain from a migraine can be so debilitating that you have to suffer time off work on a regular basis, weekends often spent in bed, sickness, diarrhea, flashing lights, loss of co-ordination, loss of use of limbs, slurring, unable to speak, double vision, throbbing pain, usually in one eye and on one side of the head, extreme sensitivity to light. Migraines do not just go away in an hour or so, and if you can't handle the pain of a headache – believe me you would be begging for mercy if you had a migraine.

It's interesting that some people are more prone to migraines than others...not everyone in the exact same circumstances will develop them. But, it seems once they start – if changes aren't made – they will continue to 'spring up' and throw a monkey wrench into whatever you have planned. Believe it or not, while there can be a number of triggers for migraines – the biggest seems to be...are you ready for this...diet. I know, surprise...surprise!!

In my clinic I've had great success offering relief from migraines by changing the diet. It's not always easy to pin down someone's specific trigger foods because there is a large list of possible culprits including foods containing tyramine (red wine, aged cheese, smoked fish, chicken livers, figs, and some beans), monosodium glutamate (MSG) or nitrates (like bacon, hot dogs, and salami). Other foods such as chocolate, nuts, peanut butter, avocado, banana, citrus, onions, dairy products, and fermented or pickled food are also known migraine magnets. Other than eliminating all of these foods or some of them for a period of time you will never know exactly what sets yours off, and it is very hard to do this on your own.

As part of my holistic approach, when I work with people on their diet, I also take into account their lifestyle, exercise, stress triggers, what food they are actually eating, hormonal disturbances and posture. That way we work on eliminating or controlling as many triggers as possible to ensure more 'migraine free' days! And, with all of my clients, I use a "clean up" plan, going through any possible lifestyle changes, learning how to deal with things in a different way, taking up exercise (even just walking or yoga) and sometimes adjustments to the posture. I think the holistic approach is best and makes you an overall healthier person. But, I have seen major improvements for people who only change their diet...because that is the biggest overall trigger. The 30 day plan in this book will certainly help.

Fatigue/Tired all the Time

Who hasn't felt tired...a long day at work, too much fun over the weekend, a few days with not enough sleep and you're tired. Usually, a day or two of 'normal' sleep and you're back in good form. But, being tired all the time...suffering from fatigue is not that simple and it's more than just occasionally wishing you could grab another five minutes of sack time when the alarm goes off. Fatigue is when your body's clock is out of rhythm and you're fighting your bodies need for sleep. Here are some of the symptoms that you fatigued men may be experiencing:

- Tired when drag yourself out of bed in the morning, feeling un-refreshed despite sleeping
- Napping in the afternoon...every afternoon
- Sleeping on the couch when you get home after work
- Unable to muster up enough energy to go for a walk, let alone to the gym, pool or play a round of golf
- Falling asleep in the car, at your desk or in meetings (not only embarrassing, but dangerous!)
- Spending the whole of the weekend in bed asleep or just too tired to get up and out
- Feeling of depression or low mood
- Loss of motivation
- Poor concentration
- Difficulty making decisions

Well, that lists makes me a little tired just writing it...and if you're actually feeling it...well, you probably just laid the book down so you could take a nap. Seriously, being that tired all the time isn't normal. So you need to look at what's going on, but guess what – it could be even worse...keep reading.

Chronic Fatigue

Chronic fatigue used to be labeled a 'fake disease." Seriously, everyone thought people were making it up, it wasn't real and that those who were suffering from CFS (Chronic Fatigue Syndrome) didn't really have anything wrong with them. Well, now we know differently. CFS is often caused by a viral illness, but often it is "the last straw the broke the camels back" in other words the sufferer has had a poor diet, lots of stress of other trigger to deal with. In my practice I see people who have become chronically fatigued through illness and because of poor diet and stress. The result is a lowered immune system leading to susceptibility of catching colds, flu and other viral illnesses which leaves the sufferer chronically fatigued, often with other symptoms such as:

- Substantial impairment in short-term memory or concentration
- Sore throat
- Tender lymph nodes
- Muscle pain - fibromyalgia
- Multi-joint pain without swelling or redness
- Headaches
- Un-refreshing sleep
- Slow recovery after exertion sometimes lasting more than 24 hours
- Unable to hold a job down
- Difficult to make decisions
- Lack of motivation

Other symptoms that may occur include:
- Abdominal pain
- Alcohol intolerance
- Bloating

- Chest pain
- Chronic cough
- Diarrhea
- Dizziness
- Dry eyes or mouth
- Earaches
- Irregular heartbeat
- Jaw pain
- Morning stiffness
- Nausea
- Night sweats
- Psychological problems, such as depression, irritability, anxiety, panic attacks
- Shortness of breath
- Skin sensations
- Tingling sensations
- Weight loss

Okay, now not only do I feel tired, but really sad. Can you imagine dealing with symptoms like this every day? Maybe you don't have to imagine it...maybe you are dealing with them. Well, there is help. But first, how do you decide you are chronically fatigued or just tired? Certainly, some of the symptoms appear on both 'Fatigued' and 'Chronic Fatigue'. But, you can look at the totality, length of time and the severity of the symptoms. If you are experiencing a number of symptoms from the first list, for "Tired all the Time/Fatigued" but not any, or many of the "Chronic Fatigue" list, then you've probably been feeling this way for no more than a few weeks (which is long enough, I know). But, if you identify with a lot of the symptoms for "Chronic Fatigue," chances are you're probably border-line or already chronically fatigued and have felt like this for some months.

Regardless of which list you identified with, neither is normal for a healthy person...let alone a Healthy Dude! So, it's time to make some changes. Certainly, you need to look at your schedule, do you have too much on your plate...too many obligations? Are you getting enough exercise? Believe it or not, taking a walk when you're tired will actually give you more energy (it's those amazing endorphins!). And there are foods that give you energy and foods that deplete your energy – especially if you're already susceptible to fatigue due to a weakened immune system. Look at some of foods to avoid for migraines...sugar, stimulants...these can cause major havoc on a tired body too. So, as much as you want that coffee and donut to wake you up...please go for some fruit and healthy protein instead. Obviously, this is just an introduction to some things to try, and, once you do go through my 30-day Detox you may be back on track. But, for a complete program, log onto www.trishastewart.com and I'll help you get your energy back for the long haul !

Weight Gain/Obesity

I know I've touched on weight issues in Chapter 3, but in case you skipped that one - thinking you eat just fine or aren't interested in my 30-Day Detox, I'm going to talk about it again. Whether you're overweight or underweight, you've got a problem that is keeping you from being the Healthy Dude you were meant to be and still could be. I'll get into both in more detail, but I'm going to start with being overweight or obese. There are HUGE health risks that every extra pound carries with it...some are literally life altering and life ending:

- High blood pressure
- High cholesterol and clogged arteries
- Stroke
- Heart disease and heart attack
- Diabetes
- Colon cancer
- Prostate enlargement and cancer
- Sleep Apnea
- Gallbladder disease
- Kidney Stones
- Sexual dysfunction

So, there are a few pleasant things to keep in mind before you bite into your next burger and fries meal combo! It may taste good, but you are potentially killing yourself or at best shortening your life. Did you also realize that being overweight increases the likelihood of depression, low self esteem, lack of confidence, anxiety, feeling like a social misfit, not being able to find clothes that fit (that can really do a number on your self-esteem). Do you seriously need more than that? Okay, then, here are some statistics I found on obesity from www.ic.nhsd.co.uk:

- 2006 – 24% of adults aged 16 or over in England were classified as obese. This represents an overall increase from 15% in 1993.
- Men and women were equally likely to be obese
- Using both BMI and waist circumference to assess risk of health problems, of men 20% were estimated to be at increased risk, 13% at high risk and 21% at very risk.
- America is home to the most obese people in the world (According to the CDC - Center for Disease Control and Prevention)
- Obesity in adults has increased by 60% within the past twenty years
- Obesity in children has tripled in the past thirty years
- A staggering 33% of American adults are obese and obesity-related deaths have climbed to more than 300,000 a year, second only to tobacco-related deaths

Wow – numbers can be fun, can't they? Look, I know it's tough. Living a life on the go, eating fast-food and microwave dinners, our health has been sacrificed. Instead of eating a diet of pure, wholesome foods coming directly from the land, most eat a diet of packaged, processed, and refined foods. Through technological advancement we have found ways to produce food in mass quantities, make it last longer and taste better. Unfortunately, during this processing somewhere along the line, we seemed to have lost the food...oops! The highly processed and refined products that pack our supermarket shelves are loaded with sugar, hydrogenated oil and plenty more ingredients that we can't even pronounce.

Fast-food restaurants have become very mainstream the past 30 years and practically all America takes advantage of the cheap prices, quick service and tasty meals. And, don't think we Brits are immune...we've got all the major fast food chains over here too, and it's not just the tourists lining up for the latest meal deal. But, convenient though they may be, these meals contain practically no nutrients. They are comprised mostly of saturated fats and highly refined carbohydrates and are loaded with sodium and sugar. One meal from Burger King, a hamburger and French fries, has 50 or more grams of fat and 2000 calories, which is almost enough to fill someone's fat and calorie quota for the day! I'm not picking on BK here...you can check out my website for links to all the fast food chains that are brave enough to list their ingredients and calories of their food items.

So, if you've got weight to lose and you're tired of the fad diets that don't work at all...or work for a bit only to have you gain more back later (we call that 'yo-yo' dieting)...then as quickly as you can start the 30-day Detox. It will set you on the path for success, you'll feel great and be looking great in no time...with more vitality and energy than you've had in ages. Trust me, the 30 day plan has worked with the "best of them". And, after the 30 days, you'll be able to customize a long-term eating plan to fit your lifestyle.

Okay, I said I'd address those who have the exact opposite problem...being underweight. It can be very frustrating to not be able to put on weight and, since most people can't fathom the problem, you get no sympathy...or support. Am I right? Well, that ends right here. There are reasons for being underweight including simply not eating enough, suffering from anorexia/bulimia, perhaps an over-active thyroid, no time to shop or cook, or over exercising and, of course, good ol' stress!. Sounds like the complete opposite of anything we have discussed above, yet there are people starving themselves to death or at best making themselves very ill though malnourishment.

One of the problems with you men is that you do not talk about these things with friends...men don't like to admit to having problems much at all, let alone a weight issue problem...especially being underweight. The focus for most men is to be big...ideally muscular, but big all the same. So, being small or thin can be a real challenge...whether it's due to a health issue, a disorder or just plain not eating enough...chances are you don't want to talk about it. Sometimes, it has nothing to do with what you'd prefer, but what your job demands. Certain professional sports such as horse racing, diving, boxing and wrestling have very specific weight categories. Men have to fall into the exact right weight range in order to qualify for the day's race, match or meet. This leads to extreme and often dangerous dieting practices...and is one of the reasons some men end up with eating disorders. Just like being overweight, excessive weight loss comes with its own set of health complaints such as:

- Decrease in muscle tissue
- Heart defects and heart muscle wastage
- Electrolyte imbalance which can lead to heart failure (salt, potassium and other tissue salts)
- Constipation
- Dehydration
- Infertility and sexual dysfunction
- Kidney stones
- Hypoglycemia
- Hypothermia
- Depression
- Untimely death

So, for any of you men reading this who are underweight, whatever the cause or reason...you can get yourself back to your Healthy Dude Ideal. The 30-Day program is a great cleanse for you and has a lot of the nutrients you may be missing. So, please give it a try. If you start losing weight...you may need to increase your portion sizes...but if you're not sure, please contact me so I can help you get an eating plan that will work for you and your specific needs.

Loss of Libido/Sexual Dysfunction

"All you need is love", sang the Beatles back in the 60's. Well that's almost right for sexual function, libido, fertility, potency and a good sex life. But it's not always quite so easy. Certainly, loss of libido can be a symptom of other problems...as you've seen in some of the health challenges I've addressed, but sexual dysfunction can sometimes be its own issue. Well, guess what, everything I've talked about so far - exercise, diet, hydration and de-stressing your life – will do wonders at maintaining a full and healthy sex life with your chosen partner.

Remember those first feelings you had as a young man...just seeing someone who attracted you? It could have been someone in school, walking down the street, or even a picture in a magazine, but you had those feelings, right? Well, you should still be having those same feelings today! That's right...because it's a chemical reaction...it's your hormones!

What happens is the eyes see, the brain connects and sends the signal to the hormonal system.

Our endocrine (hormonal) system helps maintain the steady state of our bodies. It controls our metabolism, growth and reproduction, and helps us adapt to stress and changes in our physical circumstances. It also regulates the concentrations of important substances in the blood, like glucose, calcium, sodium, potassium and water. Secreted by various endocrine glands throughout our body (and some by the neurons, or nerve cells, in our brains), our hormones act as chemical messengers. They are transported by our blood to target tissues, where they activate a change in some physiological activity. But, only if the tissue contains the right receptors. For example, for testosterone to have an effect on a particular part of our body there must be testosterone receptors awaiting its call. It's a case of needing the right key for the right lock.

Testosterone is well known for its role in the hormonal hotbed that is male puberty (remember when you started to sprout hairs and got acne). It promotes the growth of the reproductive tract, increases in the length and diameter of the penis, fully develops the prostate and scrotum and the sprouting of pubic and facial hair. As well as these androgenic or masculinising effects, testosterone also drives anabolic or tissue-building changes. These include thickening of the vocal chords, growth spurts, development of sexual libido and an increase in strength and muscle bulk. Wow, so that's how it all happens...yes...and now you know! And, these powerful physical effects continue well into adulthood.

Now, I'm not sure why, but most men think that testosterone is all there is to it; that estrogen and progesterone belong solely to women! If only it was that simple. You see, men and women produce exactly the same hormones just in different amounts. Men's bodies generate more than twenty times more testosterone than women and of course there are other hormones doing other things. So what about when it all goes wrong? What exactly is going on...or not going on? Well, unless there is a medical reason, accident or trauma there is no reason for anyone to be dysfunctional. So, that leaves three things as culprits...poor diet/hydration, poor relationship and stress.

- Stress - This stress could be in the workplace, being with the wrong partner, your living area not balanced, kids taking up all of your time, financial pressures, career move, house move, divorce, bereavement. I could go on but you get my meaning, anything that causes you stress will have a profound effect, not just on your sex life but as we have discussed earlier on your life as a whole. It just throws your entire body out of whack. So, ignoring stress and pretending things are 'fine' isn't helping anyone - least of all you.

- Relationships - Being with the wrong partner is definitely going to be a turn off. But what about when you know you really love someone, but you're just not getting that feeling you used to get? Communication is the key here. It's not always easy but unless you are able to explain your feelings or lack of them to your partner then nothing will be resolved and you'll both be miserable. Seems a few tough conversations is better than that, right? Besides it gets easier every time you talk!

- Lack of relationships - Not having a relationship can be difficult, especially if you're not feeling good about yourself. Maybe you're overweight, not toned in body or even mind, or had some of the above problems and don't feel like looking for a mate. That's ok, you don't always have to be having a full on relationship to spend time with someone. Don't get too excited, what I'm talking about is looking for a group of likeminded people and just have some fun. Remember what I said earlier - exercise and fun will release the endorphins, the happy hormones...then you'll feel better about yourself and better in general. You can also join a dating service (it's so easy to do now online) or just be very sociable and invite people to dinner, as long as they are the people you actually want to be around!!

- Diet - My favorite topic! SO much depends of what you choose to do around food. If you are going to "pig out" because you are miserable then you are going to be even more miserable later. Trust me, you'll end up with extra weight, feeling unattractive and then you'll feel worse about yourself so you'll eat more! STOP...it won't get any better this way. And, don't kid yourself it doesn't matter - it does. You really must love yourself enough first, before others will love you (except for Moms...that's why they're so great!). And, if you love yourself enough, you'll only want to put good food into your mouth. The same goes for hydration...you won't want to drink lots of empty calorie sodas and nourishment zapping coffees. You'll drink lots of water, good for you teas, healthy juices and smoothies, the occasional 'good for you' glass of wine...you get the idea. Together the right food and liquids...nourish your body, mind and soul...and your sex life!

If sorting out your diet, relationship and stress levels don't seem to be enough, then please get more help. Having a healthy libido is part of being a Healthy Dude and it's not something you have to do without. Check out Chapter 7 for some alternative therapies which will help with whatever your problem may be. It's okay to talk with someone because getting the help you need is very sexy!

Chapter 6

Tough Questions and their Answers preventing life threatening diseases.

You can set yourself up to be sick, or you can choose to stay well. **Wayne Dyer**

Guess what, it really all does come down to the choices you make for yourself. You can decide that what you do, how you live, what you eat and if you exercise are not important. Or, you can look in the mirror and realize they are. But, even that is not enough...you still have to decide what you're going to 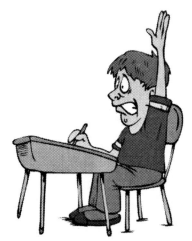 do with that information. You have to make choices about how you eat, what you drink and when you exercise based on whether you want to be the best you, the healthiest you, you can be. So, hopefully, you'll decide to live like a Healthy Dude and be on your way to optimum health. But, you probably still have one or two health concerns because of family history or too many years of poor choices in your past. I'm talking about those serious illnesses and diseases that can knock you on your butt and change your life forever. You want some answers about those things running though your mind, right? *So, what you can do to prevent and even reverse life threatening disease?*

I know – you're a guy and sometimes talking to your doctor about health concerns is harder than asking for directions, right? That's why I wrote this chapter. No one has to know what you're wondering about or what you know or don't know about health issues. And, most important, you can get the information you need to be knowledgeable, make wiser decisions and...believe it or not...prevent and often reverse some seriously life threatening diseases. Of course, I certainly can't cover everything in one chapter, but I've given you a pretty extensive look at some of the most common health issues men have to face. And, before I go on and dispense my knowledge...please remember, knowledge is NOT power...only APPLIED knowledge is power. So, if you find yourself dealing with one of these health problems and you learn what you can do to fight it...then DO IT! Take the knowledge, apply to your circumstances and rebuild...reclaim your life.

Should you be concerned with your prostate health?
Okay, let's get started with one of the biggest health concerns for men...that they most hate to discuss...the Prostate. The Prostate gland is situated just in front of and below the bladder and in front of the rectum. It produces prostatic fluid which

flows with sperm upon ejaculation. The main purpose of the prostate is to manufacture the fluid that makes up the semen ejaculated each time you have an orgasm. Sperm travels from the testicles up through a tube called the vas deferens; this joins the urethra at the level of the prostate gland where the two fluids mix and bang (so to speak), out it comes.

But, what happens when things go wrong? Well, sometimes the prostate becomes enlarged – no one is sure why – and it presses against, actually squashes, the urethra. The flow of urine is compromised and the bladder never empties properly, so there is a constant need to keep visiting the bathroom all day and night. And, spending your time in search of the nearest bathroom is no way to spend your time when you're out and about!

Here's something to remember when you're older Thomas - never pass up a bathroom, never waste a hard-on, and never trust a fart. From: The Bucket List

---

An enlarged prostate can be related to one of three conditions:

- BPH (Benign Prostate Hyperplasia) - an enlarged prostate causing irritation to the bladder and excessive urination (and in some cases reduced flow)
- Prostatitis – inflammation of the prostate
- Cancer of the prostate

Prostate cancer is the most frequently diagnosed cancer in men. Some 30,000 men in the UK alone were diagnosed with this disease, and approximately 10,000 of these men will die

(Prostate Cancer Research Centre UK 2008). Worldwide, more than 670,000 men are diagnosed with prostate cancer every year, accounting for one in nine of all new cancers in males. It is the second most common cancer in men after lung cancer.

Recent incidence rates are heavily influenced by the availability of PSA testing in the population and incidence varies far more than mortality. The highest incidence rates are in the United States and Sweden and the lowest rates are in China and India. The extremely high rate in the USA (125 per 100,000) is more than twice the reported rate in the UK (52 per 100,000). This is likely to be due to the high rates of PSA testing in the USA.

Now, having said that you should know there are many men who survive the disease. And, there are many who have cancer but don't even know it, and it's not the cancer that gets them in the end. That's because it's a slow growing cancer that often gives no or few symptoms. Some of those few symptoms that can occur in the early stages of the disease could include:

- The need to urinate more frequently
- Difficulty or pain in passing urine
- A feeling that the bladder is not empty
- Low back or pelvic pain

The frustrating thing is that, of course, any of the above could be linked to other diseases such as diabetes. Once the cancer has advanced there can be further symptoms such as:

- Weight loss
- Bone Pain
- Blood or semen in the urine

If you find you have any of these symptoms, don't ignore them...they're there to warn you that something is not right. How can you find out if your prostate is in good health or not? Well, unfortunately, one of the simplest and most common tests is the "digital" or finger inserted into the rectum test. That's why many men avoid going to the doctor to get test. However, there is also a PSA (prostate specific antigen) test, which is a blood test. And, sometimes scans may be performed for screening. Regardless of the method, if any undesirable swellings are found it is normal to be referred to a surgeon for a biopsy to test for cancer.

But take note! The best way to try and avoid this disease is to ensure that your diet is a healthy one. That means one full of antioxidants naturally present in real foods...lots of vegetables and fruit plus a high grain, bean and lentil diet. And, you should limit red meat and other flesh as much as possible due to its highly acidic nature. There are also supplements available to help with prostate health, some of which you will find on my website so please check this out and any further resource you may need. And, saving the best for last, another great tip for a healthy prostate is – use it or lose it! The more work your prostate gets the better it will continue to function.

I'm sure you're glad to hear there's yet another reason sex is good for you!

As long as I've got two of them, can I ignore my testicles?
Looks like we're going from one sensitive subject to another, doesn't it? But, this is important stuff. Unlike prostate cancer, which is prevalent in older men, testicular cancer is usually found in men from 15 - 45 years old and it affects 1 in 450 men. In the last 20 years this number has doubled with nearly 2,000 new cases diagnosed each year. While the cause is unknown, testicular cancer may be linked to men who have un-descended testicles or those with a close family history of this cancer *(Dr Rob Hicks, BBC.co.uk Health)*.

Early detection can avoid this awful disease. Just like women are asked to do monthly self exams on their breasts, examining your testicles for unusual lumps is an absolute must! Here's the truth – a lump can be the size of a pea, but if left undiagnosed it can lead to your death. I'm not saying this to scare you; just to be sure you really get how important it is for you to do a monthly self exam. By the age of 10, boys should be taught to do the simple self examination. And, if any child has un-descended testicles get this dealt with immediately as it may avoid later cancer.

The self examination should be done regularly, preferably after a bath when the scrotum (testicle sac) is relaxed. Using both hands roll each testicle gently between thumbs and fingers feeling for any lumps, swelling or unusual toughening of the sac. If there is anything unusual, contact your physician. Most often, there is nothing to worry about, but if there is, the early it is detected, the better the chance of full recovery. As a part of the treatment, it is often recommended to have the cancerous testicle removed. And, while no man wants to have the surgery, you should know it really may be the best way to ensure the cancer does not spread. Now, before you panic, read this: removal of a testicle should not affect reproduction or your sex life! In fact, it could actually save your life!

Is there anything I can do about cancer or does it just 'happen'?

Cancer is one of the most frightening diseases we'll ever have to face. I believe it's because no one really knows where it comes from. Other diseases such as heart disease and diabetes can somehow be accounted for, traced to a cause and therefore understood. Cancer is the mystery disease. Certainly, tobacco and environmental pollutions are known to cause cancer, and some people are supposed to be pre-disposed through genetics, but there are just as many cases that seem to occur without reason. There are as many as 100 or more types of cancer, all different in where they appear, how they progress and how they can be treated. They all, however, are rogue cells that can mutate the body. Cancer cells can proliferate and spread through the body systems and organs and into bone, destroying nerve cells and anything that gets in its way. While it's nearly impossible to predict if you'll ever have cancer, there are some habits and environments that increase your risk, including:

- Smoking - It may not only cause lung cancer but esophageal, mouth, larynx, pancreas and bladder cancers as well.
- Heavy Drinking – It is linked to cancers in the liver, mouth, throat and larynx.
- Poor diets – A poor diet is linked to bowel and prostate cancer.
- Sunbathing – While some sun is good for you, there is a risk of skin cancer with too much exposure, especially to those with fair skin.
- Gas Exposure – Accidental and prolonged contact with radon and other natural radioactive gases that can seep from the ground into homes and increases your likelihood of contracting some form of cancer.
- Industrial work - Workers who are subject to exposure from carcinogens such as arsenic, asbestos, benzene and other toxic chemicals are at a greater risk for some cancers.

So, what should you do, besides avoiding or limiting the above mentioned risk factors? Get checked, whether it's a self-exam or by a physician. I've already discussed prostate and testicular cancer, but here's what to look for with other cancers:

- Skin cancer – Check all moles for any changes (growth, size, color, etc.). Or, if you have a spot or sore that does not heal, and if you knock off the scab, you still bleed from it.
- Anything unusual in the urine or feces, such as blood or mucus.
- Coughing up blood
- Any unusual lump or bump that seems to have no 'cause'
- Voice box changes over a period of time such as hoarseness or a persistent cough
- Difficulty swallowing
- Fever for unknown cause
- Bad and persistent headaches
- Loss of weight and appetite
- Yellowing of the skin or even a grey tinge
- A feeling that your bones ache for no apparent reason

Remember, any of the above symptoms can be due to some other reason, so don't become obsessed. But, check in with yourself on a regular basis. Learn what's 'normal' for you and start to care about every bit of that wonderful body you have.

What can be done to prevent cancer? Well, there are no guarantees with cancer, but I promise you following an eating regime similar to what I have explained throughout this book (and my website) will lessen your chances of getting any disease. Please don't wait until 'tomorrow' to get on track, because tomorrow never comes (tomorrow is always the next day). So, start today - especially if you are not well right now! For those of you who are struggling with cancer, please visit my website for more support.

I am also an advocate of the Gerson Therapy (www.gerson.org), which you'll see is actually not too far removed from the kind of foods I would advise you to eat, but of course, less variety than you could choose in good health. Remember there is no time like the present to start; don't ever think it's too late to do anything about it; there is always something that can be done.

What the heck is diabetes anyway?
Unfortunately, more and more people are becoming familiar with diabetes because more people have it then ever before. But, I realize it may be one of those diseases that you hear about all the time, yet you don't really understand what it means or how it affects the body. So, let's start with the basics. Diabetes mellitus is a disorder characterized by the inability of the body to either produce or respond to insulin, making it impossible to maintain proper levels of glucose (sugar) in the blood. Without enough insulin (or when your body 'ignores' it) you end up with too much glucose in your blood. The excess is then excreted in the urine and that higher glucose level triggers more water flushing through. The result is

you're excessively thirsty and have to pee a lot! Those are two BIG symptoms for diabetes.

What you may not know is that there are two major types of diabetes: Type 1 (insulin-dependent) and Type 2 (non-insulin dependent). Type 1 diabetes used to be known as juvenile-onset diabetes, because it is diagnosed in children or young adults. It's caused by both genetic and environmental factors. The bottom line with Type 1 is that the person's immune system produces antibodies that destroy the cells that produce insulin. Because the body can't produce insulin on its own, daily insulin injections are required.

Type 2 diabetes is probably the type you're most familiar with. It used to be called adult-onset diabetes, because it normally appears in people aged over 40 and was quite different from the then named juvenile diabetes. But, they had to change the name because more and more children are contracting Type 2 diabetes. Why? Obesity is a major factor and, sadly, more children are becoming obese every year. The typical Western lifestyle means a diet that is high in fat and simple carbohydrates (sugars and starches), combined with little if any exercise...a sure recipe for weight issues and related diseases.

In a nutshell, Type 2 diabetes is a disorder that affects the way your body uses food for energy. Sugar from carbohydrates is digested and broken down into a simple sugar which is glucose

(Check out Chapter 3 for more details on digestion). Glucose enters the blood stream to be taken to your cells for energy. Insulin, a hormone produced by the pancreas, is secreted to help get the glucose into the cells. But, if there is no insulin or your body is not responding to it, then glucose (sugar) remains in the bloodstream and consequently you blood sugar level is too high.

It can take years to develop Type 2 diabetes, and your body can be pre-diabetic for some time. That means the body is slowly becoming insulin resistant or the pancreas is producing some but not enough insulin. At this stage you do have blood glucose levels higher than they should be, but not high enough to cause concern. That's why typically the disease shows up in people over 50...it gets worse a little at a time as a result of years of poor lifestyle choices. That's why it so alarming that this supposedly gradual disease is showing up in pre-teens. It means they're making decade's worth of bad eating and exercise habits in a few short years!

So, how can you know if you're pre-disposed to Type 2 diabetes? Here's a list of possible symptoms:

- **Frequent urination** – When there is too much glucose in the blood the body produces more urine. The lack of insulin means the kidneys cannot filter glucose back into the blood; they become overworked and try to draw more water out of the blood to dilute the glucose, making your bladder full all the time.

- **Very thirsty all of the time** – You find yourself drinking more than usual because, due to above your body becomes dehydrated.

- **Weakness and fatigue** – Glucose comes from the carbohydrates in food, insulin is supposed to help it transit into the body for energy. If the insulin is not available the carbs cannot be converted to energy, which results in tiredness and low energy.

- **Tingling or numbness in hands, legs or feet** – This type of numbness is called neuropathy and can occur over time as high glucose in the blood can damage the nervous system.

- **Other signs** – Blurred vision, dry skin, frequent infections, cuts and bruises that don't heal too well are all other symptoms that could point to diabetes.

But, there is actually good news! Type 2 diabetes (the most common) can be controlled with diet and exercise. Of course, it depends on how long this condition has been left to manifest in the body. But changes to diet and increased exercise will all help to control the problem. In fact, proper nutrition and exercise can even help Type 1 diabetics control their disease and the amount of needed insulin. That's good news, because if either type of this disease is left to its own devices, it can cause serious problems including loss of vision and amputation of limbs, as well as heart disease and death!

Why are there so many cases of heart Disease, stroke and cardiovascular problems?

If you haven't dealt with one of these issues yourself, I'm betting you know someone who has...probably in your own family. The fact that almost all of us know someone who's had a heart attack or stroke is saddening. Heart disease is truly a big, often silent, killer. In fact, the UK has one of the highest rates of death from heart disease in the world - one British adult dies from the disease every three minutes - and stroke is the country's third biggest killer, claiming 70,000 lives each year (The University of Edinburgh 2005). And, heart disease in the US claimed 869,724 lives in 2004 alone! More than 148,000 Americans were killed by CVD in 2004 were under age 65 (American Heart Society)

What exactly happens during a heart attack? It's when the blood flow through the heart is blocked, often by a blood clot. Strokes are caused either by blocked or burst blood vessels in the brain. Bottom line is that blood doesn't flow the way it should and there's an immediate STOP of movement due to the clot or burst. A stroke or heart attack can be quite mild...some people have a minor stroke and don't even realize it...or they can be deadly, sometimes immediately.

The pre-disposition or risk for heart disease and stroke may be inherited, but more often they are the result of lifestyle. Men are at higher risk for heart disease and can have attacks earlier in life. It usually affects people over 65, but it's not unheard of for men in their mid-30s to have a heart attack. It's no wonder there's an increase with the crazy busy lives most men lead...and taking care of yourself is often one of the first things set aside when things get hectic, right? So, let's take a look at some of the risky behaviors and choices that can lead to heart disease:

- **Family history (heredity)** - Children of parents with heart disease need to be more aware of their diet and lifestyle as they're genetically pre-disposed to the disease. (and have probably adopted their eating habits)
- **Smoking** - Smokers are more likely to suffer heart attacks than non-smokers, and they are more likely to die as a result. Smoking is also linked to increased risk of stroke. The nicotine and carbon monoxide in tobacco smoke severely damages the cardiovascular system.
- **Alcohol** - While some alcohol may be actually good for the cardiovascular system, drinking too much can increase the risk of heart disease and stroke because of the effect on blood pressure, weight and levels of triglycerides - a type of fat carried in the blood. Binge drinking is particularly dangerous.

- **Recreational drug abuse** - The use of drugs, particularly cocaine and those taken intravenously has been linked to heart disease and stroke. Cocaine can cause abnormal heartbeat, which can be fatal, and heroin and opiates can cause lung failure. Injecting drugs can cause an infection of your heart or blood vessels. The bottom line is that drug use brings with it a massive array of risks to your health.

- **High cholesterol** – Cholesterol levels can create a higher risk of coronary heart disease. Too much saturated fat in your diet is one cause of high cholesterol. High levels of LDL (low-density lipoprotein), or "bad cholesterol", are dangerous, while high levels of HDL (high-density lipoprotein), or "good cholesterol" lowers the risk of heart disease and stroke.

- **High blood pressure** – This may seem rather obvious, but this increases your heart's workload, causing it to enlarge and weaken over time.

- **Obesity** - People who are overweight are more likely to develop heart disease and stroke. Excess weight causes extra strain on the heart, influences blood pressure, cholesterol and levels of other blood fats - including triglycerides - and increases the risk of developing diabetes.

- **Diabetes** - Over time, diabetes can increase your risk of developing cardiovascular disease, even if glucose levels are under control. (See diabetes article)

- **Stress** - I believe there is a link between stress and coronary artery disease. Simply put, stress can encourage people to eat more, start smoking or smoke more...and those are two things that increase your risk of heart disease.

Okay, so you can't do much about the fact that your father or grandmother had heart disease, and chances are good you're doing something else that puts you at risk of having a heart attack or stroke – even if it's just having too much stress in your life. But, there are things you can do to improve your odds, including:

- Reading this book is a great start on the road to better health and longer life
- Understand the risk factors of heart disease and stroke as listed above
- Stop smoking
- Reduce your intake of saturated fats
- Reduce the amount and type of alcohol you drink (see Chap. 3 for more info)
- Increase the amount of exercise you do (see Chapter 4 for ideas and inspiration)
- Spend some time each day meditating or relaxing in some way - even if it is just lying down for 20 minutes
- Get regular blood pressure readings, height and weight monitoring and tests for cholesterol levels

The tricky thing with heart disease is many people have no idea there's a problem until they have that heart attack or stroke. That's why it's so important for you to take precautionary steps now and keep an eye on any indicators. You don't need to walk around in fear that you're about to keel over, but be smart and live wisely...so you can live better!

Am I destined to get high cholesterol?

I've mentioned high cholesterol as a lead into heart disease. But, let's take a closer look at what cholesterol is all about and why we even need it. Cholesterol is a lipid (fat) manufactured by the liver . It's present in the membrane (outer layer) of every cell in the body and insulates nerve fibers. Additionally, it's an essential building block for hormones, such as the sex hormones and the hormones of the adrenal cortex. It also enables the body to produce bile salts which aid indigestion.

Cholesterol is transported throughout the body in your blood by molecules called lipoproteins. There are several different lipoproteins, but the three main types which you're probably familiar with – LDL, HDL and Triglycerides:

- **Low Density Lipoprotein (LDL)** - While certainly necessary, LDL is often known as the bad guy due to its role in increased arterial disease. It transports the cholesterol from the liver to the cells, but too much and you can get blocking problems. And you get too much LDL – bad cholesterol – when you have too much saturated fat in your diet. Normally, the blood contains about 70% of LDL, but the level will vary from person to person.

- **High density lipoprotein (HDL)** – A little like the 'angel' and 'devil' sitting on your shoulder, HDL is the angel, or good cholesterol compared to LDL. That's because it is actually thought to prevent arterial disease. Its role is the opposite of LDL, it takes the cholesterol away from the cells and back to the liver, where it is either broken down or passed from the body as a waste product. You can see why having a higher HDL number is desired to help combat the negative side of LDL.

- **Triglycerides** - This is the third type of fatty substance present in the blood. Triglycerides are found in dairy products, meat and cooking oils, and are also produced by the liver. Fat energy from the food you eat that's not used immediately is converted to triglycerides and stored in the fat cells. However, some is also found in your blood and when the level gets too high, together with high LDL, you have an increased risk for heart disease. Those who are overweight, have a diet that is high in fatty or sugary foods, or drink a large amount of alcohol, have an increased risk of having a high triglyceride level.

The desired amount of total cholesterol in blood is under 200mg per deciliter of blood. If your number gets near 240 or above, it's too high and you need to take action to lower it. Now total cholesterol doesn't tell the entire story. Ideally, you want your LDL below 129mg/dL, your HDL around 50mg/dL and your triglycerides below 150mg/dL.

National Cholesterol Education Program Cholesterol Guidelines			
	Desirable	Borderline High	Very High Risk
Total Cholesterol	Less than 200	200 - 239	240 and higher
LDL Cholesterol (the bad cholesterol)	Less than 130	130 - 159	160 and higher
HDL Cholesterol (the good cholesterol)	50 and higher	40 - 49	Less than 40
Triglycerides	Less than 200	200 - 399	400 and higher

Evidence strongly indicates that high cholesterol levels can cause heart disease and a narrowing of the arteries (atherosclerosis), as well as heart attacks and strokes...and you've already read above how serious those can be. If other risk factors, such as high blood pressure and smoking, are present, the risk increases even more. But, once again, there are ways for you to take your cholesterol issues into your own hands and make things better. Certainly, you may find a prescription medicine to help lower cholesterol, but before you start popping those pills, first try making some lifestyle changes. Eat and exercise the right way and learn to deal with and let go of some of life's stressors. In other words, follow the

Healthy Dude plan and you'll see - things will improve and you may not need that medication.

How can I tell if I have high blood pressure or hypertension?

You've gotta have heart! Okay, I know that's cheesy, but your heartbeat is what keeps you going...keeps you alive. Your heart is a muscle that pumps a constant supply of blood around your body. First, it pumps blood that is low in oxygen to your lungs where it will receive more oxygen. Then, it pumps that blood around your body so that the oxygen can be used by your muscles and cells. Blood pressure is the measurement of the pressure exerted on the walls of your arteries as your blood moves through. There are two measurements used to assess blood pressure:

- Systolic pressure - is the blood pressure when the heart beats and forces blood around the body
- Diastolic pressure - is the blood pressure when the heart is resting between beats

Normal blood pressure is around 120 systolic and 80 diastolic, or 120/80. If your blood pressure gets into the 140/90 range...it's too high. Here's the deal...if you have high blood pressure, your heart has to work harder to pump blood around your body which, over time, can weaken it. Also, the increased pressure can damage the walls of your arteries, which can either result in a blockage, or cause the artery to split (hemorrhage). Both of these situations can cause a stroke. I know you don't want to hear this, but the number of people with high blood pressure increases with age. In fact nearly 40% of adults in England have high blood pressure.

The sneaky thing about high blood pressure is that there are really no signals or symptoms that you may have a problem. That's why it's so important to get it checked on a regular basis. Don't assume it's still fine just because it was normal five years ago, because things can change for seemingly no reason at all. So, if nothing else, next time you're at the drug store sit down at one of those free testing machines – pop your arm in the slot and hit 'go'. You may be relieved or you may decide it's time to make some changes. While slightly elevated blood pressure doesn't offer any telltale signs, that's not the case when you hit the danger zone. Very high blood pressure – that measures around 180/110 does in fact offer symptoms that include:

- A headache that lasts for several days
- Nausea
- Dizziness
- Drowsiness
- Blurred/double vision
- Nosebleeds
- Irregular heartbeat (palpitations)
- Shortness of breath

If you have these symptoms or suspect your blood pressure is to high...STOP! Put down the salt, take a break and get it checked...NOW!! There are some major risk factors that increase your chances of having or getting high blood pressure, including:

- Excessive alcohol consumption
- Poor diet
- Lack of exercise
- Obesity
- Stress

Once again, you may be tempted to go get a prescription and deal with it that way. And, in some cases you may need the extra help. But, if your blood pressure is not life threateningly high and you'd like to avoid medication, the Healthy Dude plan is for you. I know - what a surprise that I'm telling you what you eat and how you move about can fight disease and make you healthier and fitter. You may even be a little tired of hearing me say that, right? I understand...but I say it over and over again, because it's true. The right diet and proper exercise are your two biggest weapons against disease and aging. And, I'll admit that if you're way off track, getting adjusted to the program might be a bit of a struggle. But, it's so worth it when you feel strong, healthy and happy and you're disease free!

The Healthy Dude Book

So, if you haven't read through Chapter 2 and the Nine Steps to becoming a Healthy Dude flip back and give it a read. And use chapters 3 and 4 as resources for your eating and exercise plans. Don't forget that my team and I are here for you 24/7. So, if I've missed any of your health questions, you'd like further information or just feel you need some extra guidance, check out www.trishastewart.com and ask away. I truly want you to be the healthiest you can be!

Chapter 7

Alternative Help
when what you are doing ain't workin'

"People take different roads seeking fulfillment and happiness. Just because they're not on your road doesn't mean they've gotten lost." H. Jackson Brown, Jr.

Here's a big shocker...everyone isn't the same! I know...amazing, isn't it?! And, of course, now you're thinking, "Trisha – as true as that is, what in the world does that have to do with being a Healthy Dude?" Well, 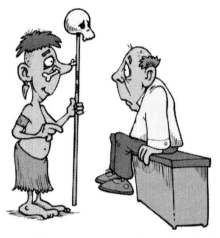 because you're different from other people, you have to find the health and fitness choices that work for you. This book is a guide for you to get on the right track, but there is more than one track that leads to Eden. So, for example, if you hate running, that's not the exercise for you...maybe you're a swimmer or a cyclist. Don't try to be a runner! And, you may need to work with a combination of approaches to get to where you want to be. It's okay if your healthy lifestyle doesn't look exactly like your friends. You may even try something that's been highly recommended, but it just doesn't work for you. So move on to something that will work for you. Are you ready for another shocker? As much as I believe (and KNOW) that your diet is the key to true, long-lasting health and vitality - I know it can't take care of everything. There, I said it.

Hold on!! That doesn't mean I want you to run off and find a prescription pill or potion or cream or shot to do the work for you. There are a number of 'alternative' treatments that can help you get to where you want to be. From head to foot, inside and out...I've created a list of these therapies, treatments and programs for you to review. I believe them all to be very effective if practiced by professional and experienced therapists and, of course, with a compliant patient. So, if you need additional support, motivation and treatment, read through the list to see which one(s) appeal to you and your unique situation. Of course, this list is by no means complete, but it's a great place to start. And, with any of the alternative methods you try, trust that each one offers help in rebalancing your body as required for you to function properly.

Many people...and you may be one of them...think therapies such as reflexology and Indian head massage are just pampering. But trust me on this, these therapies (when administered by a real pro) will have profound health benefits and help to bring about real healing. So, don't ever underestimate the power of this work.

You may notice that I have not listed any of the therapies in a "mind" or "body" category, that's because mind and body exist as "one". You'll also notice that they all seem to treat the same thing i.e. aromatherapy deals with stress and diet – so does acupuncture and even massage. I've listed more than one alternative because you need to feel it's the right choice for you and you should decide what type of treatment you want to try. For one thing, if you don't fancy needles then don't try acupuncture.

If you're sensitive to smells...skip aromatherapy. And, different people get results from different treatments. Not everyone responds to chiropractic and some get little or no relief from homeopathic remedies. So, search for what treats your challenges, go with what feels comfortable and try something else if you don't get results. However, keep in mind if any practitioner keeps you in their clinic week in week out with little or no response to treatment then something is not right, you have either chosen an incompetent practitioner or the treatment is not what you need or enough on its own or, of course, you are not patient compliant (which I know isn't the case)!

While I have years of experience, I know I cannot excel in all practices and I cannot be all things to all people. That's why I reach out to other forms of treatment for my clients. And, if anyone says to you there way is the only way...that nothing else will help...question that. Question your treatment all the way...it's YOUR health and YOUR body. Get second opinions, check with those you know and ask, ask, ask! I'm going to start out this list by explaining a bit more about my approach and the system I use. I figure it's high time you learned a bit more about me and my expertise, right?

BEST system - Me and my practice

The Scientific Approach to Health Screening The BEST (BioEnergetic Stress Testing) System represents the very latest in health screening technology. The System is fast, comprehensive and accurate. What is more, it is non-invasive and painless. There is no waiting around for the results – a detailed computer printout is available as soon as screening is completed, so both patient and practitioner know the situation immediately.

The BEST System has the ability to screen rapidly for reactions to chemicals, pesticides, heavy metals (such as the mercury in dental amalgams), bacteria, viruses, drugs, radiation, amino acids, vitamins, minerals, phenolics, hormones, alcohols, moulds, fungi, pollens, yeast, animal dander, toxins and more. It can screen hundreds of items for sensitivities under many categories. For example, it takes only 30 minutes to test for intolerance to 105 foods. Also screening for things like vitamin and mineral status or to establish whether dental fillings are leaking mercury into the body are easily carried out. The System can also be used to conduct more comprehensive screening of the entire body and its main organs such as the heart, lungs, liver and spleen.

Although based on acupuncture, the BEST System measures the points by pressing, as in acupressure, rather than the skin penetration of acupuncture needles. This is an important feature of the BEST System's non-invasive design. Using the System, the operator applies a probe to the skin surface at the acupuncture points on the client's hands (and the feet in the case of full body screening). The computer sends a very small electronic signal (5 volts @ 30 micro amps) through the skin, via the System's negative and positive contacts. The client only feels the sensation of the probe touching the skin. Readings indicating the individual's reaction are recorded by the computer as each point is measured.

The natural homeostasis of energy and temperature of a healthy human is constant. The body will always try to regulate it back to a balanced point. Just as a thermometer is used to read temperature, a highly sensitive galvanometer is used in the BEST System to monitor variations in the energy resistance of the human body. The body's bio System consists of acupuncture control points on the hands and feet - with 'control' or primary points on each meridian. A balanced reading for normal (healthy) acupuncture points is 100,000 ohms.

On the BEST System the balanced reading has been set at 50 on a scale of 1 to 100. Readings above 55 indicate an acute situation while those below 45 indicate a chronic condition. The control points indicate the overall function of say, the heart, whereas other points along the same meridian will give detailed readings - for instance, of the valves, muscles, nerves, plexus and ganglia of the heart.

A detailed report indicates the balanced, chronic and acute points relating to the various parts of the body, on both the left and right side. The practitioner can then access the 30,000 plus remedies on the BEST System to establish the most appropriate remedy needed to rebalance the points. The remedies are either homoeopathic or remedies evaluated using the homoeopathic approach (dilution's) from the many thousands of items loaded into the BEST System's memory. These items include bacteria, viruses, chemicals, homeopathics (733 main items), pesticides, sensitivities, products and many more categories. This means that the exact remedy and potency can be determined, providing dramatically improved accuracy and removing the guesswork inherent in much contemporary diagnosis.

History

In the 1950's Doctor Reinhold Voll, a Germany biophysicist, discovered a way to measure the energy level of bio-points (life-energy points used in Acupuncture) with an electrical devise. Through these measurements he could:

- Screen the energy levels of the organs in the body
- Identify toxic substances, metals, microbes, etc. that would affect the smooth   functioning of the body
- Measure food intolerance's and vitamin and mineral profile.

More importantly, he also discovered that through these same acupuncture bio-points, the effect of toxic chemicals and microbes could be minimized and corrective remedies could be identified. The major obstacle to putting Voll's work into practice was the screening method. The technique was complicated and cumbersome which meant it was too difficult for most practitioners to use in a practical and efficient way. They had to acquire large numbers of little bottles, containing the substances to be screened, if they were to carry out truly comprehensive screenings.

During the last 25 years some specialized electrodermal screening developers in USA, have been perfecting a computer system that is capable of taking these measurements quickly, simply and accurately. The substances to be tested (now numbering over 30,000) were programmed into the System and a report can be generated after each screening, showing the substances tested and the results.

Today, with the BEST System, instead of a few scribbled practitioner's notes, the client can receive a detailed personal report to take away and study at their leisure. Now, there's a lot about the system I use. If you still want more detailed information on my specific expertise (beyond the blurb on the book flap), check out my complete profile at www.trishastewart.com. I welcome your scrutiny, because as I said...it's your health...be diligent with it!

Homeopathy

Homeopathy has been used for over 200 years and was uncovered by Dr Samuel Hahnemann (1755 - 1843). Hahnemann was a German physician who was dissatisfied with the medical therapies and theories of his day. As he was translating a book by the Scot, Cullen, on medicines and their uses, Hahnemann challenged the ideas about how such medicines might work. This led him to take the substance himself so he could experience and describe its effects on a healthy human being. Repeating this type of experiment with other healthy volunteers (these experiments were called "provings") led him to observe and describe the basic principles of homeopathic medicine.

o It works on the principle that 'like treats like'. An illness is treated with a medicine which could produce similar symptoms in a healthy person.

o The active ingredients are given in highly diluted form to avoid toxicity. Homeopathic remedies are virtually 100% safe.

o Homeopathy is successful in treating a wide range of conditions, often after conventional medicine has failed.

o Homeopathic doctors use history-taking, examination and investigation.

o Prescribing is based on all aspects of a patient's condition. The patient's personality and lifestyle are important.

Heightened public awareness of the dangers of chemicals in the food chain, growing resistance to antibiotics through over-use, and concerns about the side-effects from some conventional drugs are contributing to a massive rethink about the way we live and how we seek to regain health.

Homeopathy - with its use of natural substances in minute doses, absence of harmful side-effects, and holistic and person-centered approach - is a very attractive alternative therapy.

Acupuncture and Traditional Chinese Medicine

As a great friend and colleague of my states, "it is not needle aspirin". Acupuncture is the time tested therapy that has been practiced in the Far East for thousands of years. The philosophy behind the treatment is that energy lines or meridians circulate around the body. These meridians contain our energy flow or "qi". It is when this "qi" is impaired that imbalance and illness occurs. With the insertion of fine needles at various points on the meridian, the energy can be moved or redirected to where it is needed most. In this way the body's balance can be restored and the illness resolved.

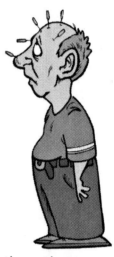

The flow of energy can be disrupted in many ways; emotional upset, physical trauma, poor diet or overwork are all common examples. By examining this underlying cause and how it has affected the body, the most appropriate treatment for the patient can be selected. Treating the patient as an individual is at the core of the acupuncture treatment and it is this that helps allow the body to rebalance itself.

Blocked energy can manifest itself in areas that are painful or are particularly cold or hot, or a different color. These signs can help determine which points are most suitable.

Western medicine often takes a more mechanistic view of people - your body may be treated as if it is a collection of machine parts rather than one whole, integrated system. Alternatively, Traditional Chinese Medicine sees individuals as personal ecosystems, with each part depending on, and influencing, all the other parts. This "whole body" approach means that treatment addresses the complete systems of your body rather than just attending to your symptoms. As a result of such a treatment strategy, most patients experience an improvement in their specific condition and also a better overall sense of health and well being. Acupuncture also includes other techniques such as cupping, moxibustion or acupressure and any of or all of these may be used.

A therapist will take a full consultation of you and your symptoms, test pulses on both wrists and check your tongue. They will then decide on the course of treatment, timelines and expected results. You may be advised to take certain Chinese herbs as part of your treatment; these should be fully explained in both their usage and what is expected from taking them.

Sports and Remedial Massage

Very useful not just as a repair mechanism when you have an injury but a good sports therapist will be able to assess muscular and skeletal imbalance and be able to put together a program of exercises as well as massage to counteract those imbalances and bring about good posture. While this form of deep massage treatment has been developed specifically to aid people suffering from injuries sustained while taking part in sports, it can be used very effectively to deal with any kind of ache or pain felt in the body since they are often caused by soft tissue dysfunction.

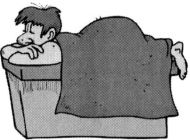

Long periods of sitting or driving can cause postural complaints which can be treated and even stress can be eased by sports massage therapy. Naturally athletes who are looking to enhance their performance and their sporting life will benefit substantially. Sports massage produces the following benefits:

- Maintains the entire body in better physical condition
- Aids cell renewal
- Removes toxic waste
- Improves flexibility
- Improves muscle tone
- Improves posture

- Alleviates muscle tension
- Helps prevent injuries
- Reduces stress and anxiety
- Improves the body's circulatory system
- Cures and restores mobility to injured muscle tissue
- Stimulates and helps to re-balance the nervous system to aid function

Sports Massage Therapy is the manipulation of soft tissue for the prevention of injuries, whist maintaining good physical condition and health. It achieves this through normalizing muscle tone, promoting relaxation, stimulating circulation and producing a therapeutically good effect on all of the body's systems.

A recommended time for allowing for recovery is usually a period of 24 hours after treatment to achieve the best effect. Additionally aftercare, such as stretching and exercise, may be prescribed to augment and re-enforce the treatment. Therapeutic oil is used as a medium. Your first consultation will provide the opportunity for the therapist to find out about your history to ensure they are fully aware of any medical or other health history that may affect treatment.

Osteopathy

Osteopathy is a way of detecting and treating damaged parts of the body such as muscles, ligaments, nerves and joints. When the body is balanced and efficient, just like a well tuned engine, it will function with the minimum of wear and tear, leaving more energy for living.

Osteopathy is a system of diagnosis and treatment which works with the structure and function of the body. The maintenance of good mechanical function is essential to good health. Problems in the framework of the body can disturb the circulatory system or nerves to any part of the body, and affect any aspect of health. Osteopaths work to restore the structure and function of the body to a state of balance and harmony, so helping the whole person.

Osteopaths consider each person as an individual. On your first visit, the osteopath will spend time taking a detailed medical history including important information about your lifestyle and diet. You will normally be asked to undress to your underwear and perform a series of simple movements. This will allow a full diagnosis and treatment plan tailored to your needs.

With their hands osteopaths identify abnormalities within the human structure and function. They then facilitate the body's ability to heal itself through a variety of stretching, mobilizing and manipulative techniques. With added exercises and health advice, osteopaths help to reduce the symptoms and improve your health and quality of life.

Your osteopath should communicate what she/he is doing so that you feel comfortable and not worrying about what they are doing. Ask questions at anytime during your consultation if you are unsure.

Cranial Osteopathy

Cranial Osteopaths view the body as a unique, interconnected, self-healing system. They believe that the structure and the function of the body are closely related, and a disturbance in the body's framework can interrupt the natural function of multiple systems, causing a wide range of symptoms. Cranial osteopathy is a specific type of extremely gentle osteopathic treatment, which focuses on relieving stress and tension throughout the body. Because it's such a gentle form of therapy, it can be practiced on people with a wide range of conditions, and is suitable for all ages, from newborns to the elderly.

Cranial osteopathy was founded by William Garner Sutherland, a pupil of the founder of osteopathy Andrew Taylor Still, in the 1930s. As a student, studying the structure and function of the human skeleton, Sutherland was particularly interested in the way the bones of the skull fit together. This fascination led him to investigate the particular structure of the skull bones and their slight malleability. It was this investigation that led to the development of cranial osteopathy and to the understanding of the role of cranial motion in health and sickness.

Cranial osteopaths are trained to feel and interpret a very delicate, rhythmic shape change that exists in all body tissues. This motion, called 'Involuntary Motion' or 'Cranial Rhythm,' comes about due to the particular movement of cerebrospinal fluid bathing the spinal cord and the pull of the soft tissue connections to the cranial bones. This involves a rhythmical elongation and narrowing, followed by a shortening and widening. This cycle repeats approximately every 10 seconds, and is separate to the rhythm generated through breathing. The motion is completely involuntary and so small in amplitude that only specially trained practitioners can feel its motion throughout the body.

Tensions and stresses throughout the body are expressed as a disruption of the body's natural cranial rhythm. As with traditional osteopathy, cranial osteopaths will perform a thorough case history and examination of their patients, however, treatment will consist of observing and treating disruptions in the cranial rhythm, whether they are due to recent events or as retained tensions due to past incidents including emotional events.

Trisha Stewart

Chiropractic

Chiropractic was invented in 1895 by Canadian-born Daniel David Palmer; a medically unqualified layman. He had been a grocer before becoming a "magnetic healer" (transferring "healing energy" to patients by touching or waving hands over them) in Burlington, Iowa, USA. He also investigated Phrenology (the belief in a relationship between the shape of a person's skull and their intelligence and personality), and he was influenced by mesmerism (a mystical healing force believed to work through hypnotic induction), spiritualism and vitalism. Vitalism is the belief in "vital energy" or a "spark of life" which distinguishes living from non-living matter; the same concept as its Chinese equivalent "chi" and its Indian equivalent "Prana".

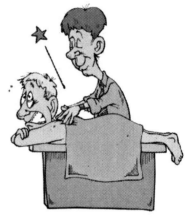

Palmer called his vital energy "Innate Intelligence". His belief was that this Innate Intelligence flowed through the body from the brain, through the spine, the nerves and on to the various organs of the body.

The theory of chiropractic which Palmer developed states that all disease is caused by the misalignment of vertebrae. A vertebra that is out of alignment, known as a "subluxation", blocks the natural flow of the vital "Innate Intelligence" through the body, thus leading to disease. Chiropractic works on the simple principle that an optimum functioning spine and nervous system equals optimum health. Good spinal alignment leads to better health and less pain.

Muscles, joints and organs of the body are controlled by the brain via the nervous system an information superhighway. Irritation of the nervous system leads to poor control of the muscles, joints and organs which in turn leads to ill health, disease and pain.

The nervous, hormonal, and immune systems are often regarded as one system. Messages are sent from the brain to other parts of the body and then back again using this "one system", with the nerve component as the master controller. The presence of a spinal misalignment called subluxations, will interfere with your body's master controller and has proven to have a negative effect on your function.

Chiropractors use their hands to adjust the joints of your spinal column, cranium and limbs where indications are that the system is compromised. This is an adjustment. Correcting these subluxations will aim to improve your body function, restore your health and reduce the pain.

Chiropractors generally treat conditions such as:

- Back pain
- Neck and Arm pain
- Sciatica
- Headaches & Migraine
- Tennis elbow/tendonitis
- Knee and hip pain
- Shoulder Problems

Colonic Irrigation or Hydrotherapy

Colonic Irrigation is safe and effective. It is a mild treatment of an internal cleansing process. It removes toxins and other burdens of putrefaction from the body, thereby assisting and supporting all other forms of natural treatment. Colonic Irrigation (colon hydrotherapy) is a well established method of cleansing the body. Dating back to ancient times, this treatment has provided an important role in relieving many health problems. By gently cleansing the colon, the body is assisted in recovering and maintaining good health. By the way, no detoxification is effective if the colon is neglected!

The world we live in is filled with substances and chemicals which are foreign and often harmful to our bodies. More importantly, the food we eat is often burdening our system with additives and agents our body cannot assimilate or handle. Our colon, also called the large intestine or bowel, is responsible for cleansing our system of solid wastes. It also provides a key role in completing the digestive process absorbing important nutrients, minerals and vitamins. If the colon is over-burdened our whole system is put under stress. An abnormal colon could be prolapsed, misshaped, affected by diverticular (pockets) and its linings could be caked up with faecal matter. Colon Hydrotherapy can help all these conditions, it assists and supports in the treatment of many health conditions and also in restoring and maintaining good health.

Herbal Medicine

Herbal Medicine is the use of plant remedies in the treatment of disease. It is the oldest form of medicine known. Our ancestors, by trial and error, found the most effective local plants to heal their illnesses. Now with the advancement of science enabling us to identify the chemical constituents within these plants, we can better understand their healing powers.

Medical Herbalists are trained in the same diagnostic skills as orthodox doctors but take a more holistic approach to illness. The underlying cause of the problem is sought and, once identified; it is this which is treated, rather than the symptoms alone. The reason for this is that treatment or suppression of symptoms will not rid the body of the disease itself. Herbalists use their remedies to restore the balance of the body thus enabling it to mobilize its own healing powers.

The first consultation will generally take at least an hour. The Herbalist will take notes on the patient's medical history and begin to build a picture of the person as a whole being. Healing is a matter of teamwork with patient, practitioner and the prescribed treatment all working together to restore the body to health. Treatment may include advice about diet and lifestyle as well as the herbal medicine. The second appointment may follow in two weeks, subsequent ones occurring monthly- this will depend on the individual herbalist, the patient and the illness concerned.

People have always relied on plants for food to nourish and sustain the body. Herbal Medicine can be seen in the same way. Plants with a particular affinity for certain organs or symptoms of the body are used to "feed" and restore health to those parts, which have become weakened. As the body is strengthened so is its power and ability to fight off disease and when balance and harmony are restored, health will be regained.

Herbal Medicine can treat almost any condition that patients might take to their doctor.

Common complaints seen by Herbalists include:
- Skin problems such as psoriasis, acne and eczema
- Digestive disorders such as peptic ulcers, colitis, irritable bowel syndrome and indigestion

- Problems involving the heart and circulation like angina, high blood pressure
- Varicose ulcers etc. can also be treated successfully
- Gynecological disorders like premenstrual syndrome and menopausal problems
- Arthritis
- Insomnia
- Stress
- Migraine and headaches
- Tonsillitis, influenza and allergic responses like hay fever and asthma

Indian Head Massage

Indian Head Massage is an effective therapy which promotes feelings of well-being and melts away tension in the body. It can be carried out seated in a chair, fully dressed, with or without massage oils. Massage is used not only on head, scalp, face and neck and shoulders but also on upper back, arms, hands and fingers, thus promoting relaxation and healing to those areas. It not only promotes hair growth but also provides relief from aches and pains. It is renowned for relieving symptoms of stress.

The effect of Indian Head Massage can last up to a week and so regular massage can bring about a sense of balance to the body and mind and restore flagging stamina.

There are many benefits to this therapy, including:

- Relaxation
- Alleviating depression
- Increasing concentration and alertness
- Revitalizes the whole body
- Improves joint movement in shoulders, arms and hands
- Aids sleep pattern
- Relief from headaches, migraine, eye strain, sinusitis and jaw ache

Initially, tiredness may be experienced after the Indian Head Massage due to release of toxins that flood the system and also to the initiation of healing energies, which require the body to rest in order to heal.

Reflexology

Reflexology is an ancient healing art and has been known to man for many thousands of years. It was first practiced by the early Indian, Chinese and Egyptian people.

Reflexology is a science that deals with the principle that there are points on the feet and hands that correspond to all of the glands, organs and parts of the body. Reflexology is a unique method of using the thumb and fingers on these reflex areas to promote the unblocking of nerve impulses in the body. This enables the body to operate at peak efficiency and aids relaxation and harmony in mind and body. Congestion, tension or pain in any part of the foot mirrors congestion, tension or pain in a corresponding part of the body.

How can reflexology help you?
The body has the ability to heal itself as I have said so many times here, but sometimes it needs a little help! Following illness, stress, injury or any disease the body is in a state of 'imbalance'. This is occasionally felt by having constantly cold feet or still lacking in energy many weeks or even months later. Reflexology can be used to restore and maintain the body's natural balance and encourage a return to natural health.

A qualified reflexologist can detect tiny congestions and imbalances in the feet and by working on these points the reflexologist can release any blockages and restore the flow of energy to the whole body. Tensions are eased and circulation and elimination is improved. This encourages the body's defenses to grow stronger at its own pace.
On your first visit the therapist will ask you various questions about your health, diet and any health problems that you may have.

The reflexologist then works on your feet, noting problem areas. There may be some discomfort in some areas, but for the most part the sensation is pleasant and soothing. The session lasts about an hour depending on your body's needs. After the first treatment you may react in a definite way: You may feel relaxed or lethargic, nauseous or tearful but this is all vital information for reflexologists, as it shows how your body is responding to treatment.

Conditions that may benefit from reflexology are:

- Asthma
- Arthritis Back problems
- Constipation
- Diabetes
- Fertility/Pregnancy
- Headaches
- High Blood Pressure
- Menstrual Problems
- Irritable Bowel Syndrome
- Menopause
- ME (Myalgic Encephalomyelitis)
- MS
- Prostate
- Sinusitis
- Stroke
- Stress

Chiropody/Podiatry

Chiropodists are highly trained foot specialists, especially when combined with Podiatry. A chiropodist works with hard skin, calluses, corns, bunions, verrucas/warts, in-growing toenails, whereas a podiatrist works with gait analysis, flat feet, heel spurs, metatarsalgia, and plantar fasciitis.

If you are experiencing lower back pain, or knee, ankle and foot pain, then it's possible that it is caused by poor foot function. Podiatrists use sophisticated analysis to determine if your gait (the way your feet work as you walk and run) is causing the problem. They will then advise and treat you. Chiropodists will determine if your foot problem is related to a disorder such as bunions or in-growing toenails.

Metatarsalgia, a common ailment treated by Podiatrists is one or more of your toe joints becoming inflamed, painful, and stiff. You may also notice swelling and experience a burning sensation in the joint area. The swelling and pain usually become progressively worse with continued activity, especially if your shoes are fairly old or you have relatively poor foot and ankle strength. In full-blown Metatarsalgia, the pain can be so intense that putting weight on your foot becomes nearly impossible.

Be aware that there are other conditions such as diabetes or gout that mimic Metatarsalgia, these must also be investigated. An x-ray - and even an MRI - might show up a stress fracture in the joint. In some extremely difficult-to-diagnose cases, tests of nerve function in the foot may be necessary.

Plantar Fasciitis - Do you have pain in your heel when you stand up for the first time in the morning? Does it feel like a knife or a pin sticking into the bottom of your foot? Then you may have plantar fasciitis. After you've been standing for a while, the pain becomes more like a dull ache. If you sit down for any length of time, the sharp pain will come back when you stand up again. Any of that ring true for you? Well, it won't go away on its own...so get professional treatment.

The plantar fascia is a band of tissue, much like a ligament, on the bottom of your foot. It works like a rope and pulley between the heel and the ball of your foot to form the arch of your foot. If the band is short, you'll have a high arch, and if it's long, you'll have a low arch, what some people call flat feet. A pad of fat in your heel covers the plantar fascia to help absorb the shock of walking.

The older you get, the plantar fascia becomes more like a rope that doesn't stretch very well. The fat pad on the heel also becomes thinner and can't absorb as much of the shock caused by walking. The extra shock damages the plantar fascia. Damage to the plantar fascia may cause it to swell, tear or bruise. You may notice a bruise on your heel or swelling in your heel.

Heel Spurs - Long standing inflammation causes the deposition of calcium at the point where the plantar fascia inserts into the heel. The result is the appearance of a sharp thorn like heel spur on x-ray. The heel spur is asymptomatic (not painful), the pain arises from the inflammation of the plantar fascia. Symptoms include a dull ache which is felt most of the time with episodes of a sharp pain in the centre of the heel or on the inside margin of the heel.

Gait Analysis – This is the dynamic assessment of the foot and lower limb with the use of high speed digital video analysis. Using high quality digital video software to capture and slow down your movements to allow in depth clinical interpretation of your movement patterns. From this the overuse injuries commonly associated with poor foot and lower limb function in both running and walking can be identified. With this information it is possible to then correct with the use of orthotic devices and physiotherapy, the underlying causes of these problems effecting long term relief of symptoms. Gait analysis is important as part of a holistic approach to the treatment of foot, ankle and leg disorders, as well as back pain and injury.

Remember what I said about looking after your feet in Chapter 2 and in Chapter 5 (don't make me bring up fungus again)? Well, this is an important part of not just looking good but creating complete harmony in body and mind.

Aromatherapy

Aromatherapy treatment draws on the healing properties of the plant world to combat digestive problems, stress related illness, pmt symptoms and more. Instead of using the whole plant it employs only its essential oil.

Aromatherapy combines these highly aromatic oils with massage, thus making use of our most primitive yet most highly evolved senses, smell and touch. Essential oils fall into many categories. Some will help physical problems, whilst others will help to address emotional needs. Even though massage is the mainstay of the art of aromatherapy treatment, these essential oils can be used in a variety of ways. A few drops can be added to the bath; they can be blended into creams and lotions for applying directly to the body, or used alone for inhaling drops placed directly onto a tissue.

Using essential oils in this way helps to promote a feeling of peace and tranquility in the recipient. In so doing, it creates favorable conditions within the Mind, Body and spirit in order that a natural balance can be restored, and energy renewed.

Treatments involve a body massage combined with a blend of essential oils that are carefully selected and diluted to suit your body's individual requirements.

Your first appointment will include a preliminary discussion before treatment begins. This is important as it will build up a picture of your present health, past medical history, dietary habits and general lifestyle. This picture will help to treat YOU, not just your presenting symptoms.

When the body is under stress, physical symptoms can occur such as:

- Digestive problems
- Stress related illness
- PMS symptoms
- Migraine/headaches
- Muscular tension
- Asthma
- Depression

Sleep can also be disturbed due to anxiety and nervous tension, and the inability to respond positively to stress can ultimately weaken the immune system, leaving the body open to viral and bacterial infection.

Aromatherapy treatment can be very helpful for pain relief and poor circulation, rheumatic aches and arthritic conditions, pre-menstrual tension and the physical and emotional stress brought on by menopause. A great number of essential oils are also very beneficial in skin care and can therefore help to balance the skin's sebum. This is very helpful for dry skin conditions.

Regular aromatherapy can help to improve posture and breathing, keeping muscle tensions at a minimum, thereby encouraging good motivation and a feeling of well being in mind and body.

Aromatherapy is especially helpful in PREGNANCY, essential oils being used from the fourth month onwards, helping with relaxation, circulation, and minor aches and pains (Always consult an aromatherapist before using essential oils in pregnancy as not all essential oils are suitable during this time) I know this book is for you guys but if you are about to become a Dad this would be a great way of helping your partner to relax and give you both some relaxing time together. So learn about these oils, just ask your aromatherapist for a blend to take home.

Reiki

Reiki [pronounced ray-kee] is a Japanese term that describes the universal life energy that flows through us all and is all around us. Universal energy is recognized by traditional forms of medicine in the East ,called 'chi' in China, 'prana' in India and 'Ki' in Japan. It is the name given to a system of natural healing which evolved in Japan from the experiences and dedication of Dr Mikao Usui who died in 1926. Dr Usui spent his life studying and researching ancient teachings and meditating on their wisdom from which he developed this healing system which he then practiced and taught to others. Reiki is still passed from master to student today. Anyone can learn or receive Reiki all you need is the desire to heal.

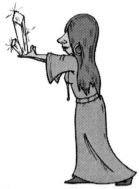

A Treatment involves lying on a couch or sitting if that is more comfortable for you, fully clothed. The practitioner gently places their hands non-intrusively in a sequence of positions which cover the whole body without actually touching it. Treatments usually last for 1hr – 1.5hrs.

Healing occurs physically, mentally, emotionally and spiritually. The practitioner is a channel which the universal energy is drawn through by a need or imbalance in the recipient. Reiki goes to where it is needed and supports the person to heal, restoring balance so that the person can regain harmony and wholeness.

Reiki is used in private practice, therapy centers, GP surgeries, hospitals, hospices, cancer support groups; post operative recovery, drug rehabilitation, prisons and HIV and AIDS centers.

Life Coach
Life Coaching is a unique relationship between you and your coach. The focus is on you, what you want in your life and what will help you achieve it. Life Coaching will take you from where you are now to where you truly want to be. You will develop

the focus, clarity and awareness you need to realize your potential. Life Coaching is an immensely powerful experience and will help you to:

- Take back control and responsibility for your life.
- Understand what is important to you.
- Identify what it is that causes conflicts and stresses.
- Create wellbeing and balance.
- Live your life on purpose and create meaningful goals.
- Regain and maintain self confidence.
- Increase Self Esteem

Your coach will listen, be curious about your goals, ask powerful questions and encourage and support you on your journey of discovery. Your coach is non judgmental, always non directive. A professional coach will offer a complimentary initial session to help you to identify the areas you wish to work on. Subsequent sessions are usually carried out on a weekly basis and the amount of sessions depends on individual requirements, some sessions may be carried out by telephone.

Hypnosis/Hypnotherapy

Within science, there is no debate as to whether hypnosis exists or works. Science simply cannot agree on what it is and how it works, although as The British Society of Clinical and Experimental Hypnosis states:

"In therapy, hypnosis usually involves the person experiencing a sense of deep relaxation with their attention narrowed down, and focused on appropriate suggestions made by the therapist."

These suggestions help people make positive changes within themselves. In a hypnotherapy session you are always in control and you are not made to do anything against your will. It is generally accepted that all hypnosis is ultimately self-hypnosis. A hypnotist merely helps to facilitate your experience and is about empowerment.

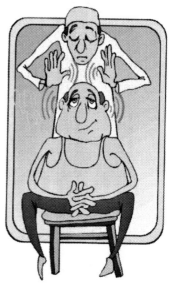

Contrary to popular belief, hypnosis is not a state of deep sleep. It does involve the induction of a trance-like condition, but when in it, the patient is actually in an enhanced state of awareness, concentrating entirely on the hypnotist's voice. In this state, the conscious mind is suppressed and the subconscious mind is revealed. The therapist is able to suggest ideas, concepts and lifestyle adaptations to the patient, the seeds of which become firmly planted.

The practice of promoting healing or positive development in any way is known as hypnotherapy. As such, hypnotherapy is a kind of psychotherapy. Hypnotherapy aims to re-program patterns of behavior within the mind, enabling irrational fears, phobias, negative thoughts and suppressed emotions to be overcome. As the body is released from conscious control during the relaxed trance-like state of hypnosis, breathing becomes slower and deeper, the pulse rate drops and the metabolic rate falls. Similar changes along nervous pathways and hormonal channels enable the sensation of pain to become less acute, and the awareness of unpleasant symptoms, such as nausea or indigestion, to be alleviated.

Hypnosis is thought to work by altering our state of consciousness in such a way that the analytical left-hand side of the brain is turned off, while the non-analytical right-hand side is made more alert. The conscious control of the mind is inhibited, and the subconscious mind awoken. Since the subconscious mind is a deeper-seated, more instinctive force than the conscious mind, this is the part which has to change for the patient's behavior and physical state to alter.

For example, a patient who consciously wants to overcome their fear of spiders may try everything they consciously can to do it, but will still fail as long as their subconscious mind retains this terror and prevents the patient from succeeding. Progress can only be made by reprogramming the subconscious so that deep-seated instincts and beliefs are abolished or altered.

What form might the treatment take? Firstly, any misconceptions a potential patient may have about hypnosis should be dispelled. The technique does not involve the patient being put into a deep sleep, and the patient cannot be made to do anything they would not ordinarily do. They remain fully aware of their surroundings and situation, and are not vulnerable to every given command of the therapist. The important thing is that the patient wants to change some behavioral habit or addiction and is highly motivated to do so. They have to want the treatment to work and must establish a good clinical rapport with the therapist in order for it to do so.

The readiness and ability of patients to be hypnotized varies considerably and hypnotherapy generally requires several sessions in order to achieve meaningful results. However the patient can learn the technique of self-hypnosis which can be practiced at home, to reinforce the usefulness of formal sessions with the therapist. This can help counter distress and anxiety-related conditions. A good therapist will give home exercises.

Hypnotherapy can be applied to many psychological, emotional and physical disorders. It is used to relieve pain in surgery and dentistry and has proved to be of benefit in obstetrics. It can shorten the delivery stage of labor and reduce the need for painkillers. It can ease the suffering of the disabled and those facing terminal illness, and it has been shown to help people to overcome addictions such as smoking and alcoholism, and to help with bulimia. Children are generally easy to hypnotize and can be helped with nocturnal enuresis (bedwetting) and chronic asthma, whilst teenagers can conquer stammering or blushing problems which can otherwise make their lives miserable.

Phobias of all kinds lend themselves well to hypnotherapy, and anyone suffering from panic attacks or obsessive/compulsive behavior, and stress-related problems like insomnia, may benefit. Conditions exacerbated by tension, such as irritable bowel syndrome, psoriasis and eczema and excessive sweating respond well, and even tinnitus and clicky jaws (tempero-mandibular joint dysfunction) can be treated by these techniques.

Cognitive Therapy

Our 'cognitive processes' are our thoughts which include our ideas, mental images, beliefs and attitudes. Cognitive therapy is based on the principle that certain ways of thinking can trigger, or 'fuel', certain health problems. For example, anxiety, depression, phobias, etc, but there are others including physical problems. The therapist helps you to understand your current thought patterns; and in particular, to identify any harmful, unhelpful, and 'false' ideas or thoughts which you have that can trigger your health problem, or make it worse. The aim is then to change your ways of thinking to avoid these ideas. Also, to help your thought patterns to be more realistic and helpful.

This aims to change any behavior that is harmful or not helpful. Various techniques are used. For example, a common unhelpful behavior is to avoid situations that can make you anxious. In some people with phobias the avoidance can become extreme and affect day-to-day life. In this situation a type of behavior therapy called 'exposure therapy' may be used. This is where you are gradually exposed more and more to feared situations. The therapist teaches you how to control anxiety and to cope when you face up to the feared situations by using deep breathing and other techniques.

Cognitive behavior therapy (CBT) is a mixture of cognitive and behavior therapies. They are often combined because how we behave often reflects how we think about certain things or situations. The emphasis on cognitive or behavior aspects of therapy can vary, depending on the condition being treated. For example, there is often more emphasis on behavior therapy when treating obsessive compulsive disorder (where repetitive compulsive actions are a main problem). On the other hand, the emphasis may be more on cognitive therapy when treating depression.

CBT has been shown to help people with various conditions - both mental health conditions and physical conditions. For example:

- Certain anxiety disorders including phobias, panic attacks and panic disorder
- Depression
- Eating disorders
- Obsessive-compulsive disorder
- Body dysmorphic disorder
- Anger
- Post-traumatic-stress disorder
- Sexual and relationship problems
- Habits such as facial tics
- Drug or alcohol abuse
- some sleep problems
- Chronic fatigue syndrome / ME
- Chronic (persistent) pain

As a rule, the more specific the problem, the more likely CBT may help. This is because it is a practical therapy which focuses on particular problems and aims to overcome them. CBT is sometimes used alone, and sometimes used in addition to medication, depending on the type and severity of the condition being treated.

The first session of therapy will usually include time for the therapist and you to develop a shared understanding of the problem. This is usually to identify how your thoughts, ideas, feelings, attitudes, and behaviors affect your day-to-day life. You should then agree a treatment plan and goals to achieve, and the number of sessions likely to be needed. Each session lasts about 50-60 minutes. Typically, a session of therapy is done once a week. Most courses of CBT last for several weeks. It is common to have 10-15 sessions, but a course of CBT can be longer or shorter, depending on the nature and severity of the condition. In some situations CBT sessions can be done by telephone.

You have to take an active part, and are given 'homework' between sessions. For example, if you have social phobia, early in the course of therapy you may be asked to keep a diary of your thoughts which occur when you become anxious before a social event. Later on you may be given homework of trying out ways of coping which you have learned during therapy.

CBT is one type of psychotherapy ('talking treatment'). Unlike other types of psychotherapy it does not involve 'talking freely', or dwell on events in your past to gain insight into your emotional state of mind. It is not a 'lie on the couch and tell all' type of therapy. CBT tends to deal with the 'here and now' - how your current thoughts and behaviors are affecting you now. It recognizes that events in your past have shaped the way that you currently think and behave. In particular, thought patterns and behaviors learned in childhood, However, CBT does not dwell on the past, but aims to find solutions to how to change your current thoughts and behaviors so that you can function better in the future. CBT is also different to counseling which is meant to be non-directive, empathic and supportive. Although the CBT therapist will offer support and empathy, the therapy has a structure, is problem-focused and practical.

Like all of these therapies, CBT does not suit everyone and it is not helpful for all conditions. You need to be committed and persistent in tackling and improving your health problem with the help of the therapist. It can be hard work. The 'homework' may be difficult and challenging. You may be taken 'out of your comfort zone' when tackling situations which cause anxiety or distress. However, many people have greatly benefited from a course of CBT

Psychotherapy

In our everyday lives we know the benefit of talking things over with friends, and sayings like "a trouble shared is a trouble halved", "getting it off your chest", and "having a good cry" bear witness to the fact that talking about and expressing our feelings helps.

Psychotherapy is a sophisticated form of this where the therapist brings to the conversation a theoretical understanding developed through formal training. An essential part of this is a long period in which the therapist undergoes therapy her/himself which helps the therapist to get a clearer self-understanding. The therapist aims to help the client identify and understand what is happening in the present in relationship to the client's background, upbringing and development so that energy available for change can be released.

People come to Psychotherapy because:

- They see destructive patterns in relationships to themselves or others
- They feel depressed and lacking purpose
- They are afraid of taking risks or making necessary changes
- They feel anxious or panicky without apparent cause
- They are experiencing a crisis
- They have experienced a traumatic event like a bereavement or accident
- They suffer from functional or psychosomatic disorders
- They want to explore and develop beyond present limits

Before embarking on psychotherapy the therapist will discuss the framework and implications with a potential client. This should be a complimentary session without any pressure to take up further treatment.

Alexander Technique

A course of lessons in the Alexander Technique will help you achieve:

- Better balance and poise
- More freedom of movement
- Relief from stiffness and pain
- More efficient use of energy

You will, look better, feel calmer and think more clearly.

Those benefits are not achieved by a system of exercises, but through a thought process that encourages awareness of how your habits of posture and muscular tension can restrict activity and impair your general well-being. Standing naturally, breathing easily and moving gracefully are activities that most healthy children take for granted, but often become more difficult as we face first the pressures of growing up and then the stresses of adult life.

In a lesson, the Alexander teacher will explain and employ gentle hands on guidance to give you the experience of freedom and lightness, which you will gradually learn to apply to more and more areas of your life. You will learn to stop what is stopping you from functioning as well as you could.

A course of Alexander lessons can lead to improvement in a wide range of problems and conditions: Back pain and other pain that does not respond to other forms of treatment;

Respiratory and digestive problems; performance-related problems for professional actors, dancers, musicians, and sportsmen...RSI and recovery from injury.

In the words of its founder, F. M. Alexander, who started teaching in London nearly 100 years ago, The Alexander Technique teaches you to make the "best use of yourself" - with mind, body and spirit working in harmony to restore and maintain optimal health.

Just scratching the surface

Well, there's just a little light reading for you to go through, right? Seriously, I put this list in the book, because I want all you awesome, amazing men to have everything you need to be your best self. It's difficult to admit you have a problem...that you need help...and it's even harder if you're not sure what kind of help you need. This is an introduction to some alternative therapies and treatment styles I fully endorse. They're all safe and real, but they're not all going to be a fit for you. But be brave and check one of two of them out. Even if you don't need something more intense like Cognitive Therapy, I'm betting you could use something that helps you relax and distress a little...so try an Indian Head Massage or some aromatherapy. And, if you can manage, ask a trusted friend for advice on what to try. The best way to find a therapist or form of therapy is by referral from a friend. And, since I'm your friend now as well, you can always contact me.

Maybe you need more details about a certain type of therapy or treatment...well log onto the website and contact me. The answer may be right there on the site, but if it isn't...I'll do my best to find it for you. Remember, ask questions and seek answers!

Afterword

Well, if you've made it through this book, then you've got some great information to start your new Healthy Dude lifestyle. And, if you're one of those who likes to sneak a peak at the back of the book to see how it ends...here's the punch line: yes, you can transform yourself into the Healthy Dude you'd like to be!

Sure, it's going to take some work...you will have to change the way you eat (some of you more so than others), make real exercise a part of your daily life, learn to deal with stress (because we all have it), get rest, practice good hygiene and – most importantly – have the right attitude. But, by following the '9 steps' along with the eating and exercise plans I've laid out in this book...it will happen.

But here's the most important thing I want you to take away from reading this book...good health and a vibrant life are within your reach and I'm here to help you attain both! Whether you're just a little out of shape and need to get back on track or you're dealing with some major health challenges, together we can address your unique situation and get the results you deserve. So, please, if you need more support, have questions or are looking for more information, visit my website www.TrishaStewart.com and start searching. From new recipes and workout routines to the latest research on men's healthy...it's all there.